From Both Sides of the Curtain

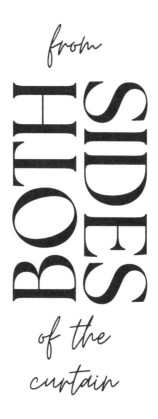

from

BOTH SIDES

of the

curtain

LESSONS AND REFLECTIONS
FROM AN ONCOLOGIST'S PERSONAL
BREAST CANCER JOURNEY

SUE HWANG, MD

NEW YORK

LONDON • NASHVILLE • MELBOURNE • VANCOUVER • BOSTON

From Both Sides of the Curtain

Lessons and Reflections from a Oncologist's Personal Breast Cancer Journey

© 2025 Sue Hwang, MD

Published in New York, New York, by Morgan James Publishing. Morgan James is a trademark of Morgan James, LLC. www.MorganJamesPublishing.com

Proudly distributed by Publishers Group West®

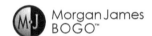

ISBN 9781636987910 paperback
ISBN 9781636987927 ebook
Library of Congress Control Number:
2025938601

Interior Design by:
Chris Treccani
www.3dogcreative.net

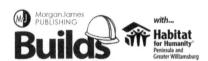

Morgan James is a proud partner of Habitat for Humanity Peninsula and Greater Williamsburg. Partners in building since 2006.

Get involved today! Visit: www.morgan-james-publishing.com/giving-back

To my mother, father and sister, who laid a solid foundation from which I could thrive with grace.

To my three sons, who gave me the strength to get through every day.

To my awesome circle, who embraced me and my boys as one of your own.

To my amazing village, who showered my family with love and unconditional support without us ever needing to ask.

To my doctors, who stood by me through every step of my treatment and beyond.

And to my patients, who taught me that we all deserve better.

Contents

Acknowledgments

Thank you to Dave Cobb for putting this book writing idea in my head and giving me the confidence to do it.

Thank you to Mary Hayes, Kristen Edsall, Kat Pick, Tracy Kelly, and Almira Torralba for their invaluable time and effort in editing this manuscript.

Thank you to Scorpions Baseball Academy, Canes Florida Baseball, Bishop Moore Catholic School, and Orangewood Christian School for supporting my children through all they have been through. You went above and beyond without me asking and I will be forever grateful.

Thank you to Jessica Burdg for guiding me through the book writing process.

Thank you to Bronwyn Stall, Lisa Minton, Dave Kawczynski, and Joe Ciaramella for capturing the soul of the book through its cover.

Thank you to Morgan James Publishing for believing in this project and supporting me in my first endeavor.

Introduction

"Five minutes!" I scream, my voice echoing throughout the house in our typical morning chaos. This is my daily signal that sets three boys, three dogs, and one overwhelmed radiation oncologist into the final morning motions. My oldest son starts loading his iPad in his backpack. My middle finally emerges from his room after his third wake-up call. My youngest heads to the sink and grabs his toothbrush. Meanwhile, I'm orchestrating a complex dance of filling water bottles and mentally running through my day's schedule while also trying to sequester a four-year-old Boston terrier who still hasn't mastered the art of potty training, a six-year-old Italian mastiff who counter surfs when left unsupervised, and a thirteen-year-old pit mix who rivals Oscar the Grouch's affinity for garbage.

This is—*was*—my normal: a carefully calibrated routine where every minute counts. Drop-off at three different schools, a work schedule where I was often double or triple booked, administrative meetings, baseball games and practices, and somehow a home-cooked dinner on the table at the end of the evening. I took pride in being a single working mom and one of the top producers in my medical practice. Sure, I was treading water most days, but I was treading water successfully. At least that's what everyone told me.

"You really have it all together," they'd say. On the outside, maybe I did. But inside? Inside, I was emotionally and physically exhausted, running myself ragged, postponing joy and pushing toward some future moment when things would finally slow down.

That future arrived sooner than I expected, but not in the way I had hoped.

THE DAY EVERYTHING CHANGED

What stands out most about that Wednesday morning was the normalcy of it all. It was my administrative day, the one day a week I could wear yoga pants and a sweatshirt instead of my usual white coat. I sat in a dimly lit room with chairs lined up against the wall, half-watching HGTV while waiting for my colleague Tim to read my routine mammogram.

As a radiation oncologist specializing in the treatment of breast cancer, I'd spent fifteen years guiding women through this exact moment. I knew the drill: get your mammogram, wait for the radiologist's review, and then head back to your regularly scheduled life. When the tech said Tim wanted to see me in his office, I wasn't concerned. As a professional courtesy, he always showed me my images. When he told me that he wanted more imaging, I still wasn't particularly concerned because I knew he was thorough.

But then I saw Tim's posture—head hanging with his glasses sliding down his nose and thumb pressed against his temple and forefinger against his forehead. He couldn't meet my eyes. In that moment, before he even spoke, my brain shifted from "just another Wednesday" mode to something else entirely.

"The ultrasound showed five masses in your breast," he said quietly. "And there's a lymph node that looks a little abnormal."

The room tilted sideways. As a doctor, I knew exactly what this meant—the number of masses, the lymph node involvement, all of it suggesting an aggressive cancer that had developed frighteningly fast over the past year. I could barely breathe.

Within hours, I went from being Dr. Hwang, a confident and successful radiation oncologist, to a terrified patient holding onto her best friend while getting a biopsy. And somehow, amid this blur of scans and tears, all I could think was *I'm going to be late for my car dent repair appointment that I've waited two months for.*

Looking back now, I have to laugh at that detail—how the mind clings to the ordinary as everything else is falling apart. But that's the thing about cancer: It doesn't care about your carefully scheduled life, that you're a doctor who treats cancer, or that your kids need you. It transports you to an alternate universe where your life is temporarily halted even though the world around you keeps spinning. It just shows up, uninvited, and redefines everything you thought you knew—even when you thought you knew everything there was to know about breast cancer.

WHY THIS BOOK

I never intended to write this book. As a doctor, I'm used to being the one with answers, the one who guides others through their cancer journey. Being on the other side of that equation wasn't part of my plan.

But sometimes the most important stories are the ones we never planned to tell.

This book is both a memoir and a mirror—not only reflecting on my journey from doctor to patient and back again but also illuminating the complex emotional landscape that every cancer patient must navigate. It's about what happens when medical knowledge meets lived experience, when clinical expertise collides with raw human fear.

Through these pages, I'll take you with me through each step of my journey—from the shock of the diagnosis, through surgery, chemotherapy, and radiation, and then into the strange new world of survivorship. You'll see cancer treatment from both sides of the medical curtain: the doctor who understands the science behind every treatment and the patient who becomes paralyzed with every little pain.

But this is more than just a story of an oncologist's cancer journey. It's also a story about resilience, about finding strength in vulnerability, and about the unexpected gifts and moments of levity that can emerge from our deepest challenges. It's about learning to live fully in the present when the future feels uncertain and about finding humor in the darkest moments (trust me, they exist). It's about remembering that the patient is a person who has needs and concerns beyond eradicating the disease. Most importantly, it's a story about hope. Not the simple kind that promises everything will be okay but the complex, mature hope that acknowledges fear while refusing to be defined by it.

Whether you're a patient seeking understanding, a caregiver looking for insight, or a healthcare provider wanting to better understand the patient experience, I hope you'll find something valuable in these pages. Because while cancer may be a medical condition, healing is a human experience—one that requires both scientific knowledge and emotional wisdom and I want to speak about both. As a doctor and patient, I've learned there's a significant gap between knowing medical information and truly understanding what it means for your life, and the only way I was able to bridge this gap was to stand on both sides of the curtain myself.

Welcome to my story. I'm glad you're here.

Chapter One

WHEN DOCTOR
BECOMES PATIENT

The mammography waiting room always played HGTV. I'd been in this space countless times before—having started routine screening at the age of forty. I always booked the first appointment of the day because I knew all too well how easily schedules could get backed up. Like clockwork, the tech called my name soon after I checked in, and within minutes my breasts were being pressed between two plates of the X-ray machine. Once she had obtained all the necessary images, she directed me to wait in a holding room while Tim, the breast radiologist and a longtime colleague, looked at my images. She returned a few moments later and led me to his office, which was hardly concerning because he always reviewed my scans with me. What was concerning? That he couldn't meet my eyes.

"You have a new area of calcifications in the upper outer quadrant of your right breast. It wasn't there last year," he informed me as he pointed to a large number of scattered white dots of varying shapes and sizes on the computer monitor.

I reviewed the images and agreed. "Yes, I see them. Well, at least there aren't any masses," I sighed with relief, as I assumed the irregular calcifications were likely ductal carcinoma in situ, aka Stage 0 breast cancer, which is easily treatable.

"No definite masses," he agreed. "But there is an area of asymmetry. We need to do an ultrasound to get a better look."

The warm ultrasound gel on my breast felt jarring against the cold air of the exam room. I tried not to look at the screen, tried not to interpret the clicking sounds of the tech capturing images or the silence that followed each measurement. But fifteen years as a radiation oncologist made it impossible not to understand exactly what was happening.

That's when he delivered the news: five masses in my breast, the largest being three point six centimeters, and an abnormal lymph node too.

My world fell out of focus for a moment. Three point six centimeters echoed in my head. *How did I not feel something that big?* My doctor's brain immediately started predicting tumor biology and calculating growth rates while my mother's heart seized with panic. *What about my boys?*

FROM PROFESSIONAL TO PERSONAL

I was moved to the hallway of the radiology department, where I sat while they prepped the room for a biopsy. As I was trying to process what was happening, one of the techs approached.

"Your patients love you so much. They also talk about how nice you are. I'm sorry this is happening," she said softly. "Can I give you a hug?"

I wanted to scream. Nice? I didn't want to be nice. Nice people died. I'd seen it too many times in my own practice—the kindest patients, the ones who never complained and were more concerned with others even as they suffered through their own treatment. They were the ones who broke my heart.

Instead, I found myself nodding, accepting her hug.

"This is so unfair," she continued. "You help so many women."

I nodded again, not knowing what to say. I knew there was no such thing as fair, especially when it came to cancer.

I needed to talk to Devina. She was one of my best friends, my sister in everything but blood, and one of the busiest breast surgeons in Central Florida. We first met when she interviewed with the medical group for an open breast surgeon position. During our hour-long one-on-one meeting, we talked about everything but the job. Her oldest son was the same age as my youngest, and we decided they would go to school together and be friends. We picked the neighborhood her family would move into and established that she would get along well with my circle of friends. When she accepted the position and relocated to Florida, all that we predicted came true, and our families grew into one big extended family.

Devina, at five feet tall, was small but mighty. She had no problem calling people out and holding them accountable for their actions. One year, when we decided to host the annual office holiday party at an upscale steakhouse, the service was uncharacteristically bad. Halfway through the event, she left the table to find the manager. "Excuse me," she said after she tapped him on the shoulder. "Can you tell me what restaurant we are at?" He looked at her, confused. As he opened his mouth to respond, she interrupted him. "Because I made a reservation at Christner's. But it doesn't feel like I'm at Christner's. Christner's is known for their exceptional service, which I have yet to see tonight, so I wanted to make sure we were at the right restaurant." And just like that, the service improved dramatically . . . and all cocktails and desserts were comped at the end of the night.

I knew Devina was upstairs in the hospital operating all day, but maybe I could catch her in between cases. My hands shook as I dialed her number. When the OR nurse answered, I cleared my throat and tried to keep my voice steady.

"Is Dr. McCray available?"

"I'm in a case right now," Devina called out, her voice distant on speakerphone. "What do you need?"

"There's something wrong with my mammogram." I could barely get out the words.

"What do you mean?" Her voice sharpened.

"They found five tumors." The sob caught in my throat. "And a lymph node."

"Get her off speaker!" Devina barked. Then, directly in my ear: "Where are you?"

"Downstairs, in the radiology department."

"It's going to be okay."

"It's not going to be okay, Devina!" I snapped back.

I could hear her directing her team to finish up, as she promised to come find me. Within minutes, my colleagues were transformed into my caregivers. Wassim, a close friend and breast medical oncologist, placed orders for a battery of tests. He sent his nurse, Chassidy, to keep me company as I waited for insurance to approve the biopsy. She was a quiet guardian who worked in almost every department and knew almost everyone in the hospital. If I needed anything, she would know exactly who to call. When the ultrasound suite was ready, she gave my hand a tight squeeze and mouthed, *It will be okay.*

Once I laid down on the table, I heard a snap as the nurse broke open a chlorhexidine stick and applied the cold antiseptic to the surface of my breast. Tim entered the room, barely recognizable in his mask and scrub cap. "Let's begin the time-out," he said professionally. His need to verify my identity prior to the procedure made me acutely aware that I was no longer a colleague. "This is Sue Hwang. We will biopsy two masses in the right breast and a lymph node."

Just then I heard Devina in the hallway. She knocked quietly and entered the room. By this time, the first mass was visualized on the large screen overhead. Devina took one look at the screen and said nothing. She grabbed a stool, sat down by my head, and started running her fingers through my hair. "It will be okay," she whispered in my ear. "It's probably nothing." But I knew from the tears running down her cheeks that she knew this was cancer. The professional demeanor I'd maintained for fifteen years crumbled in an instant. I was no longer Dr. Hwang, the confident oncologist. I was just another scared patient, watching my whole world shift on what should have been a routine Wednesday morning.

THE VIEW FROM THE OTHER SIDE

In oncology, stage dictates treatment. The moment Tim mentioned a suspicious lymph node, my brain started racing through different treatment algorithms—neoadjuvant chemotherapy, axillary dissection, postmastectomy radiation. Each possibility carried its own set of toxicities and complications. Each decision point represented another way my life would change.

A three point six centimeter mass developing between annual screenings meant the tumor was growly quickly. Multiple tumors scattered through the lateral aspect of my breast meant I would need a mastectomy. An abnormal lymph node meant that the cancer was one step closer to spreading to other parts of my body.

"I need a full body scan," I insisted after the biopsies were completed. "Right now."

Devina tried reasoning with me. "You just had the biopsy. Let's wait for the results—"

"We both know this is cancer. There's no question after looking at the images." I waited for Devina to disagree, but she fell silent. "I need to know if it has spread. Three point six centimeters is huge and I didn't feel it at all! How did I not feel it? What else is growing in my body that I don't know about?" These words caught in my throat.

There was conveniently an opening on the CT schedule from a last-minute cancellation, so we walked down the hallway to the scanner. The tech directed us to a holding area as she finished up with another patient. Just then, Devina's husband, Q, appeared. Q worked as a reporter/anchor for the local ABC affiliate. He clearly came straight from work, as he was still wearing his navy-blue polo with WFTV embroidered on the upper left chest. In addition to having a comforting presence that made it easy for anyone to open up to him, he had no fear, which allowed him to knock on the doors of suspected murderers to obtain exclusive interviews. He also had a soothing voice and a calming demeanor, which was exactly what I needed before going in for a scan that would tell me if the cancer had spread.

"I have to go back to surgery, and Chassidy had to go back to work, so I called Q," she explained. "I don't want you to be alone. I'll call you when I'm done operating." And she disappeared down the hallway.

"Well, this is not how I saw today going," I joked as he awkwardly laughed. Just then, the tech announced she was ready for me.

Q stood watch as my entire body slid in and out of a machine. I lay perfectly still on the cold, hard table, trying not to think about how many times I'd ordered these same scans for my patients. Images of bones and lungs filled with cancer flashed before my eyes. Once the scan was completed and the whirring of the machine stopped, Devina shouted from the control room, "I don't see any cancer anywhere else in your body. No mets, Sue. No mets! Okay, now I really have to go."

Then she was gone again, rushing back to surgery, leaving me with Q, who asked gently if I wanted to go home.

"Actually," I said, "I have a dent repair appointment for my car. Can you go with me to drop it off and drive me home?"

"PATIENT NAME, PLEASE."

"I need you to come to my office now," Wassim, who naturally fell into the role as *my* medical oncologist, commanded over the phone as Q and I drove back from the car repair shop. "We need to order genetic testing. I also want to order genomic testing to get an idea of if you need chemo . . . and basic labs because I don't see anything recent in the system. Out of curiosity, when was the last time you saw a doctor?"

The truth was I couldn't remember the last time I'd seen a doctor—as a patient, that is. Devina ordered my yearly mammograms, another friend performed my pap smears, and I didn't have any health concerns. If there was ever an acute issue, I would "phone a friend" and ask them for their professional advice. I knew this wasn't ideal, but I didn't have much spare time for a routine doctor's appointment. My kids, my job, the dogs, folding the laundry, getting dinner on the table—those all took priority over a wellness visit with a primary care physician.

When I got to Wassim's office, his normally talkative staff fell silent.

"Guess what happened to me today?" I exclaimed. They all looked at me with a half-smile. No one knew what to say.

"Doc, let's go in here so I can get some blood," Amy, a medical assistant whom I'd worked with for the past six years, said as she stood up and directed me into an open exam room. "Have a seat while I grab some supplies." She closed the door behind her and I reflexively sat down on the doctor's stool. I'd been in this room countless times before, meeting patients with newly diagnosed breast cancer. The stool was always reserved for the providers while the patient would sit on the exam table and family members would sit in the chairs. But today, I wasn't the doctor and Amy would need the stool as she drew my blood. Recognizing this, I got up and moved over to the exam table. As I waited for Amy to return, I stared at the now empty stool.

"You know we need your signature to run the tests." She handed me a clipboard with a stack of consent forms. After I finished signing, she asked me, "Patient name, please." I looked at her with a raised eyebrow. Was she being serious? "Sorry, Doc," she apologized. "Standard procedure."

"Sue Hwang," I responded. And with that, she drew several tubes of blood and patched the puncture site up with a bandage.

"Stop by the boss's office before you leave," Amy instructed. "He wants to talk to you."

Wassim's door was open, and I could hear him typing away on his computer as I approached. When I peeked my head into his office, he stopped what he was doing, laid his glasses on the desk, and stood up with open arms. I leaned in, and he gave me a tight hug. "It'll be okay," he said. "I talked to the pathologist already.

They are waiting for the biopsy and will process it as soon as they get it."

"It's cancer, isn't it?" I asked, already knowing the answer.

He nodded. "It is. Tim knew just by looking at it."

Wassim was always honest about what he was thinking. While there was still a little part of me holding out until the biopsy came back, Wassim was grounded in reality and charging forward with a plan. Patients appreciated his candor, almost as much as they appreciated his good looks. I always got a good laugh whenever mutual patients shared completely inappropriate fantasies about him. But on a serious note, he was a fierce advocate for those he took care of and stayed connected with every doctor on the care team so that he was always well informed.

"You know the drill as well as I do. Receptor status and genomic testing will drive our decision-making. Now we wait . . ." His voice trailed off because we both knew that waiting for results was the hardest part.

I wandered next door to my office to gather a few things before heading home. Marie, the lead radiation therapist and mother hen of the department, found me in my office. "What are you doing here? Isn't it Wednesday?" she questioned, knowing that I usually worked from home on Wednesdays.

"It is, but I got my mammogram this morning." I sat down in my chair and debated about telling her. But then I figured she would eventually find out. "It didn't look good. I think I'm going to need some time off work."

She looked at me for a moment, then the questions started: "Are you sure it's right?"

I explained that we had only just done the biopsy, but it looked like cancer. Marie just nodded and shifted immediately into problem-solving mode: "Okay. Whatever you need, just let me know.

Want me to figure out coverage? What about the kids? Grocery shopping? The dogs?"

I didn't have any answers. I was still stuck in the surreal space between diagnosis and acceptance.

"I don't know" was all I could say.

THE DENIAL PHASE

The next morning, I woke up convinced it had all been a mistake. The embarrassment hit hard—I'd already told Marie I had cancer and got the wheels turning for treatment. What if I'd overreacted?

"It's probably from Zeus," I told Devina over the phone. My one hundred and eighty-five pound Italian mastiff was always forgetting his size, crushing whatever—or whoever—was in his path when he got excited. "It's probably just trauma from when he stepped on my breast as he was trying to climb onto the bed."

Devina, bless her, played along. "Could be," she said, though we both knew better.

I started my day seeing patients in the morning. Over the lunch hour, I participated in the weekly breast tumor board, which was a meeting where all the breast cancer specialists meet to discuss complex cases. As I looked up at the screen, I listened to the radiologist review the PET scan of a newly diagnosed thirty-six-year-old female with metastatic breast cancer in her lung, liver, and bones. One of my colleagues sighed, "This poor woman." I wondered what comments they would make about my case if I were presented.

It was a challenge to focus on the discussion as I waited for my own results. The sound of the seconds ticking away was deafening in my ears. The waiting felt endless. How many times had I told patients "These things take time" without truly understanding the agony of those words?

After the meeting I returned to my office and attempted to complete paperwork. Then I saw Wassim and Devina appear in my doorway together, and I knew. The pathology was back.

"It's an invasive lobular cancer," Wassim said quietly. "It's estrogen and progesterone receptor positive and HER2 negative."

The tears started before he finished speaking. I hated lobulars—they're sneaky and can spread without obvious signs. Devina knelt beside my desk, hugging me while I cried.

"We're taking you to surgery next week," she said firmly. "I've already talked to Sabrina about reconstruction. She made room for you on her schedule. She'll do the case with me."

I started to nod, then froze. "What about the lymph node?"

Wassim stepped out to call the pathologist. When he returned, his face said everything.

"It's positive."

And just like that, I officially went from being a cancer doctor to a cancer patient.

THE PATH FORWARD

The three of us sat shocked in my office, trying to register all the results. Lobular. Multicentric. Lymph node positive. Each finding by itself was serious enough, but to have all three together? I stared at the patient charts on my desk. My name would soon be on similar forms, but not as the signing physician. The thought made me nauseous.

Cyndi, my nurse practitioner, knocked gently. "You have patients waiting."

"Cancel them," Devina instructed from beside my desk. "Cancel the rest of the day."

But I couldn't cancel everything. Life doesn't stop for cancer. I still had to take care of my boys. I still had to take care of my patients. The real challenge wasn't just processing my diagnosis— it was figuring out how to keep living and maintaining normalcy for those around me.

My first step would be telling those I loved . . . starting with my kids. James, at fifteen years old, had already had several friends lose their mothers this past year. The causes were all different, but the end result was another friend without a mother. Sam was no different, having one friend's mom pass from cancer and another friend's father die in a car accident. And Nathan, the youngest, had been asking increasingly pointed questions about death lately. "What happens when you die? Will it be dark forever? What does eternity feel like? It seems scary."

The boys had watched their friends navigate that impossible terrain of death. Now here I was, about to tell them they might be stepping onto that same path. How do I tell my children I have cancer when all I want to do as their mother is protect them from the harsh realities of the real world?

The irony wasn't lost on me. Part of my job as an oncologist was to help patients navigate this difficult discussion with family and offer advice about how to break the difficult news. I would always tell patients to be as open as they were comfortable being and to be honest. It's better to deflect a question than to lie because children know when someone is lying. Now, sitting in my office with mascara streaking down my cheeks, all that professional wisdom felt worthless.

Devina squeezed my hand. "One step at a time," she said softly. "We can tell the kids together. They're stronger than you think."

I nodded, trying to believe her. But as I caught a glimpse of myself in the window reflection, I didn't see Dr. Hwang anymore.

I saw what my patients must see when they first get their diagnosis—someone whose life had just split into "before" and "after," frozen in fear in that space between.

"YOU ARE NOT A NUMBER"

As a radiation oncologist, I explain biopsy results to patients on a daily basis. But nothing prepares you to go through your own results.

"Lobular," Wassim had said. My stomach dropped. Most breast cancers are ductal, which develop in the milk ducts and form a mass that can be easily seen on mammograms or ultrasound. Lobular breast cancers are different. They're sneakier, starting in the lobules of the breast, aka the glands that produce the milk, and growing in single lines. Medically, the term is "Indian filing" because it resembles the way that Native Americans walked along a trail. Their growth pattern can make them difficult to detect on physical exams, as was the case in my situation, and on imaging.

Lymph node involvement changed everything. In medical terms, it meant my cancer was at least Stage IIB. In personal terms, it meant a more aggressive treatment plan because the cancer had already made its way into my lymphatic system. In emotional terms, it meant the thing I'd feared most as a doctor, losing control of my body, was now my reality as a patient.

I turned to my computer to review studies that I knew like the back of my hand; except now I wasn't looking at the data from the perspective of a supervising doctor, but rather a mother who was desperately trying to predict how much time she had left with her children. What percentage of those patients had lobular cancer? What percentage had lymph node positive disease? What percentage had more than one tumor? How many were locally controlled at ten years? How many were still alive? I devoured the data like a starving person, searching for certainty in a suddenly uncertain world.

Wassim caught me. "Stop looking at that," he said firmly, closing my laptop. "You are not a number."

But I was. I was multiple numbers now: forty-six years old, five tumors, one positive node, three point six centimeters. These figures would follow me through every step of treatment, markers of my new identity as a cancer patient.

ONE DAY AT A TIME

The next few days passed in a blur. My initial surgery date was pushed back a few days because Wassim wanted more imaging.

"You need a PET," he urged. "The CT scan showed a really small lung nodule. It's probably nothing, but there is a lot of cancer in the breast, and you have a positive lymph node. We need to make sure you don't have metastatic disease."

I knew he was right, but I didn't really want to do the scan on the small chance that something would show up. I preferred to live obliviously in peace rather than apprehensively in reality. A week ago, my biggest stress was Sam not handing in his homework on time. Now my biggest stress was whether I'd be alive to see him graduate from high school. Every twinge, every slight pain now carried new weight. Was that shoulder ache from overdoing it or had the cancer spread to my bones? The doctor in me knew this was irrational but the patient in me couldn't stop obsessively worrying.

In addition to more imaging, I needed an official consultation with Sabrina, a friend, colleague, and well-respected reconstructive breast surgeon. She completed her training at an Ivy League school and her impressive surgical skills were only outmatched by her gracious bedside manner. She was also a perfectionist, something I'd always appreciated when referring patients to her. Now that perfectionism would be focused on me.

"We'll do a nipple lift on the left," she announced, studying my chest with professional detachment. "You're a little saggy on that side. We want perfect symmetry when this is done."

I wanted to laugh. Perfect symmetry? I just wanted this cancer out. "I don't care what my nipples look like," I told her. "Just take them off."

"No, no," Sabrina insisted. "Let me do this for you." I could only nod in silent defeat.

The photos were next—clinical shots from every angle, measuring and marking with surgical precision. This was standard procedure, I knew that. But standing there in front of the camera, arms raised in various positions while my colleague documented my "before" state, stripped away any remaining pretense that this was just another medical procedure.

After the pictures, she went into full-blown doctor mode.

"You don't have enough tissue for flap reconstruction, so I recommend we go straight to implants," she explained. "This way we can get everything done in one surgery. Silicone is the best option for patients undergoing mastectomy. The texture is similar to natural breast tissue, and it moves better with your body. They also last a long time."

She pulled out several implants of varying sizes. "Do you want to go bigger?" she asked with wide eyes and a huge smile as she held out two ridiculously large implants.

I laughed. I knew she was doing her best to lighten up a serious situation. I guess the one benefit to this diagnosis was the option to size up while getting insurance to foot the bill.

"No," I said, shaking my head. "I just want what I have now. I don't want to have to buy different clothes."

"That makes sense," she said in agreement. "The implants will be placed on top of your muscle. It will be wrapped in AlloDerm, which is human cadaver skin. The AlloDerm acts like Velcro, holding the implant in place. I will make you look great!"

"Now let's talk about how to minimize lymphedema," she continued. "We're going see how things look intraoperatively before we commit to aggressive lymph node surgery. If we have to go that route, then I'll perform a lymphovenous bypass. By rerouting the cut lymphatics to the veins in your arm, we can reduce the risk of arm swelling by fifty percent."

"One more thing and then we are done. As you know, Devina and I are starting to perform breast neurotization." I remembered Devina talking to me about this new technique. She and Sabrina had flown to New Orleans to take a course on how to preserve nipple sensation for women undergoing mastectomies. They performed their first case several weeks ago, and I was guessing I would be their second.

Quite honestly, retaining sensation in my nipples was the last thing on my mind. But I knew they could only perfect the technique by performing it, so I agreed to be a willing participant. She continued, "Postmastectomy numbness is a huge complaint from patients, so we're hoping this new technique can help restore sensation. Devina will find and preserve the nerves as much as possible, and then I'll use a nerve graft to reconnect what has been cut. It can take a few years to know if it was successful."

It was interesting to learn about the reconstruction process firsthand. Breast cancer management has become so specialized that, while I understood the basics of what my fellow doctors did, I did not keep up on the specifics. When asked questions outside of my specialty, I gave general answers and deferred more thorough explanations to that specialist. Because cancer requires a multidisciplinary approach, I explained that it was important for doctors to "stay in their lane" to minimize confusion. That said, there were so many nuances to the other specialties that it wasn't possible for me to provide detailed answers confidently.

As I left Sabrina's office, I called Tracy, one of my best friends who lived in Wisconsin. We met after we'd both just graduated from residency and were hired by the Medical College of Wisconsin to staff a satellite clinic in Kenosha, a city located north of the Illinois–Wisconsin border. We instantly bonded over the anxiety and stress that came with managing patients independently without the safety net of a supervising physician overseeing our every decision. We talked about anything and everything and it didn't take us long to develop a sisterly bond. I blamed her for introducing me to the mastiff breed, which I found incredibly endearing despite all their slobber and flatulence issues.

When I left Wisconsin for a better job opportunity in Florida, she joined me on the three-day road trip and never got annoyed at Nathan, who would only stop crying if he heard the opening scene from Frozen, which we were forced to play over and over and over again. Despite the distance, we continued to talk almost daily on our way to work, bouncing interesting cases back and forth, venting about children, or simply catching each other up on life. She was a fiercely loyal friend who I could always lean on for support and guidance during my tough times. And despite having a family of her own as well as a demanding job as a breast radiation oncologist, she insisted on being by my side when I underwent the mastectomies.

"I'll be there on Sunday night," she said. "I'll Uber, so you don't have to worry about getting me at the airport."

"If you are going to take time off of work and be away from your family to help me through surgery, then I am going to pick you up at the airport," I insisted.

"Or you can just buy me another mastiff," she joked. "Just kidding. Okay, I'll see you at the airport. You doing okay?"

Reality was hitting me hard. In a few days, Tracy would be here and I would be undergoing surgery. I was silent for a few seconds. "I'm scared." That was all I could say, trying my best to hold back the tears.

"I know," she responded quietly. "I'm here for you. Take this one day at a time."

But the future rushed toward me like an oncoming train, and I hadn't told my family yet. Despite all the treatment that lay ahead, I knew telling my family would be the hardest part of all.

Later that night, I sat in bed reviewing my images on my laptop—so many masses that had somehow grown undetected in my breast. The largest one mocked me. *How had I not felt the tumor? I'm trained to find these things in others. How had I failed to find them in myself?*

Zeus rested his head on my lap, his weight anchoring me to the present moment. The medical knowledge that had defined my career now felt like both a blessing and curse. I understood too much to take comfort in platitudes yet somehow not enough to protect myself from this disease. I closed my laptop and laid down. As Zeus snuggled up beside me, I realized this journey would require more than just my clinical expertise. It would demand everything I had—as a doctor, a single mother, and a woman facing her own mortality.

In the morning, I would have the hardest conversation of all: telling my children their mother had cancer. But first, I needed to find the strength to say those words aloud myself.

"I have breast cancer."

The words hung in the dark room, heavy with implications.

I said it again. "I have breast cancer."

It was real now. There was no going back to before.

There was only forward.

Chapter Two

BREAKING THE NEWS

Today is the day. I have to tell them. I have to tell them. The thought had been running through my head on repeat, like a broken record. Now here I was, sitting in the passenger seat of James' Hyundai Sonata—a car I purchased for him a few months shy of his sixteenth birthday. When he got his permit, I taught him how to drive in my behemoth GMC Yukon XL. As testing day for his driver's license drew near, I wanted him to get used to driving something other than my school bus. I gave him a budget and after some research he announced that he wanted a Hyundai Sonata.

"A what?" I questioned, surprised that he wanted a four-door sedan and not something . . . cooler. But that was James, always practical and economical. He was frighteningly intelligent, highly self-motivated, and extremely confident. He wasn't bothered by other people's opinions because his self-confidence came from an innate understanding of who he was.

As I sat next to him, I struggled to figure out the best way break the news. James was talking about baseball as he always did, and I wasn't even pretending to listen, too preoccupied with rehearsing the words in my head. Since I counsel patients for a living about how to have difficult conversations with their families, I thought this would have come more naturally. But there I was, unable to find the best words to tell my child about the diagnosis.

Not knowing how to start the discussion, I finally just blurted out: "I have cancer."

James stopped mid-sentence, and his hands stayed steady on the wheel at ten and two just as he had learned in drivers ed. "What?"

"I have breast cancer," I elaborated, watching his profile carefully. "Ms. Devina is taking me to surgery on Friday, and I'll be down for a few weeks."

He didn't say anything at first, just stared straight ahead at the road, but I could see him processing. His face remained still, but his eyes gave him away. Then came the quiet sniffles he was trying so hard to hold back, followed by the tears he couldn't quite contain.

"James, I'm going to be okay," I said, falling into my doctor voice without meaning to. "Ms. Devina will be doing the surgery, and—" I paused to think of what more I could say to reassure him when he cut in.

"How long have you known?"

"I just found out two days ago," I answered.

He nodded slightly, still focused on driving. I waited for him to say more, knowing the context he was carrying: one friend's mom gone from metastatic breast cancer, another from a stroke, and a third from chronic illness. The weight of that knowledge hung heavily in the car between us.

Finally, James spoke again, "How do you know you'll be fine?" he questioned. His voice thick but carrying that characteristic dry wit that made him uniquely him. "No offense, Mom, but you guys are kind of dropping like flies."

I couldn't help but laugh, even as my heart ached. Trust my too-smart-for-his-own-good fifteen-year-old to find a way to interject humor in the moment. For the next few minutes, I answered his questions as directly as I could, treating him almost like a patient's family member—which, in that moment, he was. How bad was it? What kind of surgery? Would I need chemo? What about radiation?

It wasn't the perfect way to tell him. But then again, is there ever a perfect way to tell my child I have cancer? Sometimes the most authentic moments come when we least expect them, even if they happen when my inexperienced teen driver is driving fifty miles an hour down the road. In retrospect, telling my son that I have breast cancer while he was operating heavy machinery was probably not one of my best parenting decisions. But there was something about having him focused on the road ahead that made it feel . . . safer, somehow.

TIME TO DO HOMEWORK

After we got home, I knew I had to tell Sam next. As expected, he was in his room, shades drawn and lights off, doing what most thirteen-year-old boys love to do—playing Fortnite. "Sam, can you please shut that off? We need to talk." Something in my tone must have gotten through because asking a teenager to stop playing video games typically requires at least ten attempts and then a threat. This time, however, he sensed something was off. He simply said, "Okay" and quickly turned off his computer.

He sat next to me and silently waited for me to talk. Sam is my child who processes everything internally. He was seven when his father and I announced we were getting divorced. Unlike James, who knew it was coming and quickly verbalized his thoughts on the matter, Sam sat on the couch almost in a trance, unable to say a word. His normally expressive face went blank, and I could tell he was thinking about the change that lay ahead. A minute later, his tears started flowing, and he let out an agonizing cry. It broke me to see his heart ache and to know I was the reason. And at that moment, I vowed to do everything in my power to never cause him that much pain again. Now, as I prepared to find the right words, I knew that I would have to break that vow I'd made to myself so many years ago.

"Hey, Sam," I said gently, grabbing his hand in mine. "Mom had a test last week that shows I have breast cancer."

Silence.

"Ms. Devina is going to take me to surgery on Friday," I continued. "I'll be down for a few weeks, but I should be back on my feet in no time. I'm going to be okay. I know this is scary to hear, but I'm going to be okay."

Silence. No tears.

"This is what I do every day, and my friends will take really good care of me." I was running out of things to say but couldn't bear the sound of silence, so I rambled on. I would have been okay with tears at this point because his lack of verbal and emotional response made me wonder if he was even listening.

I was about to ask him if he was okay when he pulled out his cell phone and started typing away.

Oh my God, I thought to myself. *I'm telling my child I have cancer, and he's texting? WTF!*

Before I could express my frustration, he looked up at me and said, "I'm doing my math homework."

And with that one explanation, I knew that he'd heard and understood what I'd said.

Sam, unlike his older brother, does not have a proclivity for school. He does, however, have an extremely high level of emotional intelligence and knows how to read a room and respond appropriately. This makes him extremely likeable and naturally the center of attention. His desire to socialize, unfortunately, often interfered with his ability to do schoolwork in a timely fashion. To keep him on track, I would constantly remind him to do his homework. These reminders eventually turned into a lecture on the importance of handing in assignments on time and doing well in school. And when that didn't register, I inevitably ended up pleading, "Please, just do your homework to make Mom feel better."

His response was his way of showing me that he'd take stress off me by doing what I was always asking him to do. While James needed information and facts, Sam needed to feel useful. He couldn't fix the cancer, but he could do his homework without being asked. It wasn't the reaction I was expecting, but the more I thought about it, it was classic Sam, and he brought me so much comfort without ever having to verbally acknowledge the cancer.

SO MANY QUESTIONS

Nathan was a different story entirely. At eleven, he didn't personally know anyone who'd died and barely had a concept of what cancer was. While he knew I was a cancer doctor, he understood the job to be one that paid Mom well so that he could live in a big house and buy expensive baseball bats. Then one day, a few weeks before my diagnosis, he came home from school and told me that one of his teachers was very sad because his father was just diagnosed with cancer.

"Mom why is he so sad?" he asked. "You treat cancer patients all the time, and you don't come home sad."

"Cancer is scary for a lot of people," I explained. "And it's different being the doctor that treats cancer. Mom's job is to try to get rid of it, but sometimes you can't get rid of it." Little did I know that a few short weeks later, I would be telling him that I had cancer.

I was so emotionally drained from talking to James and Sam that I can't recall the exact words I used. But I do remember his response. There were no tears, just questions.

"Are you going to die?" he asked immediately. When I said no, that this was caught early, he pressed harder: "Can you promise me that you aren't going to die? What will happen to me if you die? How do you know you're not going to die? You said it can be hard to get rid of."

Then he pressed on with more difficult questions. "What does death feel like? Is it dark forever? What does it mean to live forever in heaven? Does that get boring? Is it the same day over and over? I don't understand this feeling of forever." Such difficult questions that I never would have anticipated my eleven-year-old asking.

There were no good answers to his questions. As a doctor, I could cite statistics and survival rates. As a mother, I wanted to promise him everything would be fine, but I knew that was a guarantee that was out of my control. Instead, I had to sit with his fear, acknowledge it, and be as honest as I could: "I don't know for sure, but I do know this was caught early, and this is what Mom does for a living. A lot of patients do well with treatment. We just have to take this one day at a time, okay?"

That answer didn't satisfy him then, and in some ways, it still doesn't. While he was on the cusp of entering the teenage years, he still looked to me for guidance, support, and approval. News of my diagnosis crushed whatever innocence remained, opening his eyes to the existence of a harsh reality where everything isn't always rainbows and butterflies.

In response, Nathan developed a hypervigilance over my whereabouts, tracking my every move like a worried parent:

"Where are you going? What time will you be back? Call me when you get there." When I traveled for conferences or took James on college visits, he monitored the flight tracker and asked me to call him before I took off and as soon as I landed. Sometimes he demanded to come along, and other times, he begged me not to leave. He was love-stalking me, as I came to think of it—his way of trying to keep me safe through sheer force of will.

Each of my boys processed the news differently because they each needed different things from me. James, at fifteen, needed facts and control. Sam, at thirteen, needed practical ways to help. Nathan, at eleven, needed reassurance that his world wasn't about to fall apart. As their mother, I wanted to protect them from anything that could hurt them. But I knew that wasn't possible—or even necessarily helpful. Sometimes the best thing we can do for our children isn't to shield them from hard truths but to show them how to face reality with courage and honesty, even when we are really scared ourselves.

A LEGACY OF STRENGTH

In the 1950s, my mother was one of the only women in her medical school class in Taiwan, following in the footsteps of her mother—a pioneering midwife whose portrait hangs in a museum for delivering more babies than anyone else in her region. I am honored to share a legacy of strong women that I'm only now beginning to fully appreciate. After her husband died young, my grandmother built an impressive life for herself. While caring for three young children, she accumulated wealth, invested in the local university, and embodied the mentality that "if you work hard, you'll succeed."

My mother brought that same drive with her when she came alone to the United States in the late 1960s. Already a doctor in

Taiwan, she had to complete another residency in New Jersey and chose obstetrics and gynecology. She opened her own solo practice and was on-call 24/7, with her after-hours schedule dictated by whenever the babies decided it was time to enter the world. She was a no-nonsense doctor who didn't sugarcoat things for her patients. I remember one time when we were having dinner at home, she received an emergency page from her patient. From what I gathered, the patient recently underwent a hysterectomy and started bleeding heavily. "Did you have intercourse recently?" my mom asked. When the patient didn't answer, she asked again, a little bit louder. The patient must have said yes because my mom started half lecturing, half shouting, "What did I tell you about intercourse after surgery?" She waved one hand in the air before smacking her forehead in frustration. "No intercourse, no sex for the first six weeks after surgery. Go to the emergency room now. I will meet you there." She grabbed her car keys and slammed the door behind her.

Despite the grueling on-call hours and a busy, all-consuming practice, she still somehow managed to serve a home-cooked dinner every evening. She also focused heavily on investing in our education. But as much as she was there for us, she also held us to exceptionally high standards. For her, education wasn't just important, it was everything. My sister and I weren't expected to just go to college; we were expected to go to medical school. She made tiger moms seem like pussycats. She was a pioneer for the independent working woman who somehow managed to do it all. Following in her footsteps was an incredibly challenging task that at times seemed impossible.

My father was also a doctor, not the MD kind but rather the PhD kind. He grew up in the Taiwanese countryside during World War II and would tell stories about having nothing but rice to eat because the army marched into town and took "all the good stuff". Because of this, we were never allowed to waste any food in our house. He eventually earned the nickname "the human garbage disposal", eating all leftovers before consuming anything freshly prepared. He was so poor growing up that when he boarded a boat from Taiwan to Japan, where he went to further his education, he brought a suitcase of bananas to sell onboard to make some money.

Eventually, he made his way to the University of Wisconsin, where he earned a PhD in biochemistry despite speaking very little English. He often recalled how he never had any friends until it got closer to exams, at which time classmates would surface from every direction asking for his notes or help understanding the material. Once he graduated, he moved to New Jersey to work for a chemical supplies company, and it was in New Jersey where he met my mom.

But his story then took an unexpected turn when my sister, eighteen months my senior, and I entered the picture. Apparently, we were not easy children and had a revolving door of nannies. Eventually, he quit his job to care for us and opened up a home business selling baskets. Yes, baskets. He used our three-car garage as his storage room, leaving no room for cars. To this day, he still hasn't given me a great explanation for how he went from a PhD-holding biochemist to a basket seller, but the latter is how I'll always remember him.

In what was progressive for their time, my father was the stay-at-home parent. He was there when my sister and I got home from school, helped with homework, drove us to our after-school activities, and dropped us off at our friend's house for playdates. In an era when most of my friends' mothers were ever-present, mine was in a hospital, working all hours of the day and making most of the household's financial decisions. It was different, but it worked.

THE WEIGHT OF SACRIFICE

Even though my parents worked hard and built a financially secure life, my father still lives as if he has nothing. He continues to wear clothes that were handsewn by his mother seventy-five years ago. He places empty plastic containers under the bathtub faucet to collect whatever drips out because that water can be used for the plants. He never throws anything out if it still has a function. When I was a child, he would fish out of the garbage can half-used pencils that my sister and I threw away.

My mother is no different. She recalls walking to school as a child with no shoes. She still wears my tattered West Essex High School Tennis team shirt like it is perfectly good clothing—because "it is". She saved and lived frugally so my sister and I could go to college and medical school without loans. And once we completed our education, she started saving for her grandchildren so they could go to school without loans. On our annual family ski vacations to Telluride, we all sported matching ski wear from brands like The North Face and Patagonia. My mother, on the other hand, would wander out in three layers of pants, a teal-colored winter coat and a fluorescent pink and yellow fleece hat that I wore as a child.

My parents instilled a strong work ethic in me and are the reason I am the person I am today; their steadfast guidance shaped my values, teaching me that dedication, perseverance, and integrity are the keys to achieving my goals. However, our relationship isn't the kind where I can confide all my worries and concerns in them. As they moved through life, saving every penny and investing in our futures, they did so with an eye for survival and a penchant for caution.

This history of sacrifice and success made telling them about my diagnosis especially complex. My mother lives in a state of perpetual fear and paranoia. She watches the evening news religiously and draws dire conclusions about the world: "You can't go out at night because that's when most people die." "Don't let your kids go to sleepovers because they can get molested." "Don't meet people over the internet because they just want to scam you or rape you."

I understand now that her fear comes from survival. When so much of your early life was dependent on making it and building something from nothing, you see danger everywhere. For these reasons, our relationship exists in this space between deep gratitude and perpetual tension. While I understood the magnitude of her sacrifices, I struggled against the weight of her expectations. It's a dynamic that shaped how I approached telling her about my diagnosis because the generational gap between my mother and me isn't just about years—it's also about worlds. In her world, there's constant overcast with a dense, oppressive layer of storm clouds always rolling through whereas in my world, the skies are typically blue and the sun is always shining.

After my diagnosis, I wondered: How do you tell the people who sacrificed everything to give you a perfect life that perfection isn't possible? Sometimes the hardest part of being a child of immigrants isn't living up to their expectations—it's figuring out how to disappoint them gently.

THE NEWS GETS OUT

My solution to telling my parents about my diagnosis was . . . well, not to tell them. At least not right away. My sister, Min, and I had a long conversation about this. She is a breast radiologist who practices in Arizona and having informed thousands of her patients of their cancer diagnoses, she knows firsthand how stressful this news would be on our parents. Min was always the smarter, harder-working daughter and, in my mind, the favorite. She was valedictorian of her high school class and granted admission to the honors program in medical education at Northwestern University, which guaranteed her a spot in their medical school right out of high school so long as she didn't totally slack off in college. Even though I towered over her five-foot two-inch body, I always felt like I was living in her shadow. When it came time to decide where to go to medical school, Northwestern was my obvious choice, since attending the same school would finally show my parents that I was just as good as her.

"Let's just wait," she said over the phone. "Better to disclose when we have the whole picture. Telling them you have cancer and then waiting for results will be agonizing for them." I knew she was right. Our mom was eighty-five, and our father was eighty-nine, with ninety only a few short weeks away. On a good day, mom's anxiety was already through the roof. Why add to that? Dad, on the other hand, lived every day happily oblivious as he entered a time of senility, so who was I to ruin that? Min and I thought we could handle everything quietly, get through surgery, and then tell them when we knew the exact stage of the cancer and confirmed what further treatment would be needed.

But life had other plans. Specifically, life had my soon-to-be ex-brother-in-law, who learned of my diagnosis through mutual friends and took it upon himself to tell my mother without my knowledge.

So there I was, getting an unexpected call from my mom: "How's your health?"

The casual tone didn't fool me. My stomach dropped. "What do you mean?"

"A little birdie told me you're having surgery."

I was going to kill my brother-in-law. Actually, I was going to let my sister kill him first, and then I'd kill whatever was left. I knew it was him because he called me right before my mother, insisting I tell her. We'd argued about it for thirty minutes before I ended the call, firmly stating I wasn't ready. I was so angry that he took that decision away from me.

There was no way to get out of this one, so I spilled the beans. Yes, I had breast cancer. Yes, I needed surgery. I downplayed the number of tumors and didn't emphasize the involved lymph node. I kept repeating what an incredible team I had and offered a phone call from every doctor that would be taking care of me if that would make her feel better. "I do this every day, Mom," I remember saying. "I'm not worried," I lied. "I don't want you to worry. I know exactly what's going to happen. Everything is going to be fine. Do you have any questions?"

"Just one," she replied. "Who's going to wipe your butt?" And with that question, I knew she understood what was going on and had shifted into "practical" mode.

"What kind of question is that?" I said in disbelief.

"Sue, you aren't going to be able to move your arms very much after the procedure. Have you thought about that at all?" I knew she was right, and, no, I hadn't thought about it.

"Mom, I'll figure that out when the time comes. I have to go," I said, trying to get off the phone because I was horrified at what other bodily function she would tell me I needed help with next.

"One more thing," she interjected before I hung up. "Don't tell your father. He's almost ninety. He doesn't need this stress, and he won't understand."

That's my mother—simultaneously showing deep concern and trying to shield my father from worry while probably spiraling internally. In that moment, I could see all the layers of our relationship: the cultural expectations, the generational differences, the medical knowledge we both carried, and the eternal dynamic of mothers and daughters trying to protect each other in their own imperfect ways.

It wasn't how I wanted her to find out. But maybe there is no good way to tell your mother you have cancer, especially when she's spent her whole life trying to protect you. Sometimes the best we can do is accept the messy reality of family dynamics and try to navigate them with as much grace as we can muster.

THE WORD STARTS SPREADING

The dynamics in a medical office are unique. As the doctor, you're at the top of the hierarchy, with staff working under you. But cancer has a way of restructuring everything, including professional relationships. My fellow doctors were immediately supportive: "Whatever you need. Tell us what you need. Time off? Fine. Need us to see these patients? Fine."

Initially, I only told my immediate colleagues, keeping it quiet from the rest of the staff. Then they knew something was going on when I was out of the office until further notice.

Marie approached me again: "What do you want me to tell the staff? Right now, we're just saying there was an emergency."

I hesitated. "I don't know."

"Well, we need to tell them something."

Finally, I said, "Whatever, just tell them I have breast cancer."

After that, the food started arriving at my house daily. Casseroles, Mexican food, Chinese food, Olive Garden, Cracker Barrel—so much Cracker Barrel.

Naturally, the "doctor out for the foreseeable future" message sparked concern among my patients. Some who'd known me for years started texting. One message in particular touched me: "I just want you to know your office is doing a really good job of respecting your privacy. I don't know what's going on, but I hope whatever it is, you will be on the mend soon. I missed seeing you today. No need to respond." Others simply wrote: "Not sure what happened, but we're thinking about you." It was overwhelming to receive so many messages, and they all reminded me of just how lucky I was to be in so many people's thoughts.

I also found myself being profoundly humbled when I became a patient in my own hospital, having the hospital staff care for me in a completely different way. My relationships with my colleagues deepened. The staff who'd always looked to me for direction now supported me in ways that had nothing to do with medical hierarchy. The boundaries between my professional and personal life, already blurry to begin with, became almost nonexistent.

Medicine has never been a nine-to-five job. We give our cell phone numbers to patients who need them, and answer texts and calls outside of normal office hours. In addition, I commonly run into patients when I'm out and about, most of the time while doing errands—and one memorable time in a dimly lit bar, just after midnight, while trying to find my way to the bathroom. Regardless of the venue, patients would often take these chance encounters to ask questions that were on their minds, and I'd always take the time to answer them, even when I *really* had to go to the bathroom.

As physicians, we spend a fair amount of personal time discussing complex cases with each other. Because most of the working day is consumed with seeing scheduled patients, squeezing in urgent consults, and documenting in a timely fashion, patient care is often coordinated during personal time. While establishing clear work boundaries sounds amazing in theory, it's not practical, especially when time is of the essence. Cancer doesn't stop growing on the weekends or when the doctor is on vacation. It's almost considered normal to have personal time interrupted to ensure that everyone is on the same page when it comes to patient care.

While I grew accustomed to being perpetually "on the job" to some degree, it was impossible not to think about breast cancer every waking moment now that I was straddling both sides simultaneously—the caregiver and the cared-for, the professional and the patient. There was no respite from the diagnosis, no safe place I could hide to take a break from my new reality. It's a perspective I never wanted but sometimes the most profound insights come from being forced to walk in your patients' shoes.

THE ART OF BEING VULNERABLE

I learned to wear different masks for different audiences. With my kids, I'm strong but honest. With my patients, I'm professionally distant yet personally understanding. With my colleagues, I'm medically precise. With my mother, I'm selective with information and protective even as I seek protection. Each conversation requires a different version of myself, a different balance of truth and hope.

Being a doctor who specializes in the very disease you're diagnosed with creates its own peculiar challenges. You understand the medical language but struggle to translate it into emotional reality. You've said "You'll get through this" to countless patients, but now you're learning how hollow those words can feel when you're the one hearing them.

During this time, I felt the professional identity I'd built over the years begin to crumble. How do you maintain authority in your field when you're also vulnerable? How do you counsel patients about their fears when you're grappling with your own? These questions would follow me as I began treatment, forcing me to reconstruct not just my body but my understanding of what it means to be both healer and patient.

If there's one thing I've learned from sharing my diagnosis, it's that vulnerability isn't weakness—it's connection. Every time I opened up about my diagnosis, whether to my children or my colleagues, it created a bridge. Sometimes that bridge carried support and love my way. Sometimes it reminded me how we all face different struggles, even when we all seem so put together on the outside.

Sharing my diagnosis allowed others to share back, others whom I never would have suspected of having a history of cancer—like one of the partners in my medical practice, several years my junior. I called him to get an opinion on a complex case, and at the end of our conversation, he confided that he knew what I was going through. "When I was in my twenties, I was diagnosed with testicular cancer," he said. "Then I also found out I had lymphoma in my skin." I was shocked. He was so young, so optimistic, so healthy now . . . not someone I would have expected to have a history of one, let alone two cancers.

A few days later, Aimee, the COO of the hospital, stopped by my office. "You WILL get through this," she said confidently. "You are strong." I looked at her and thought, *Easy for you to say*. She was the epitome of a boss lady. She was able to cut through the hospital politics that had become all too common at big institutions and advocate effectively for her physicians. Before her, I was used to administrators who deferred complicated issues until they were promoted to their next position in the system. She, on the other hand, wasn't here to passively climb the ladder, she was here to get results. She was a no-nonsense leader who was kicking butt and taking names along the way—all while looking amazing in a leather suit jacket and four-inch heels.

She was able to sense my doubt and removed her glasses. "Look at me." She leaned in. "Do you see this?" She removed her glasses and pointed to a subtle crease along her right cheek.

"Is that a wrinkle?" I asked as I squinted to get a better look.

"No, it's a scar from where I had a melanoma removed several years ago. It was a huge surgery, and they had to take part of my forehead and move it down to my cheek to cover the big hole that was left when they removed the cancer." She explained it all surprisingly nonchalantly. "I know you're scared, and I know the treatment won't be easy. But I also know you'll get through this, and I'm here for you, whatever you need." She said it so convincingly that it was hard not to believe her. I didn't respond. I just sat at my desk, staring at her face.

As others found out about my diagnosis, I learned of even more health struggles that friends and co-workers privately battled. In every instance, after I got over the shock, I took comfort in knowing that I wasn't alone. I soon realized that everyone will be faced with something at some point in their lives and these challenges will shape and define who we are. Not talking about these things outwardly doesn't mean that they don't affect us inwardly. The masks we all wear—doctor, mother, daughter, patient—they're not fake. They're all real parts of who we are. The trick is learning when to let them drop so that others can see the fear behind the strength, the uncertainty behind the knowledge, and the humanity within us all.

I used to consider my independence a badge of honor, amazing so many onlookers with my ability to successfully manage single parenting while holding down a full-time, high-demand job. But adding breast cancer to the mix made it impossible for me to keep doing everything by myself. I was already treading water on a daily basis, looking calm and collected on the surface but wildly flailing all my limbs below just to stay afloat. Breast cancer added a hundred-pound weight to my shoulders that made it impossible to continue keeping my head above water, and the only way to survive was to rely on others for support. Needing others in this manner was such an uncomfortable, unsettling feeling, but cancer forced me out of my comfort zone of independence.

As I prepared to undergo surgery, I knew I needed others to help me maintain some semblance of a normal life for my kids. Being openly vulnerable was one of the harder parts of my diagnosis. But I had to take a crash course on letting others in with surgery only days away. I learned quickly that strength doesn't always look like independence. Sometimes it looks like letting your teenager drive while you tell him difficult news. Sometimes it looks like accepting casseroles from colleagues or letting your son do his homework instead of talking about his feelings.

This was just the beginning of the journey, but already it was teaching me lessons I never expected—about family, about medicine, about strength, and about the complicated dance between helping others and accepting help myself. The masks we wear might change, but the face beneath them—vulnerable, scared, determined, loving—that's the one that matters most.

Chapter Three

WHEN IT GETS REAL

There's something surreal about picking up one of your best friends from the airport so she can help you through cancer surgery. Tracy and I had been through a lot together—new babies, career transitions, cross-country moves, and my divorce. She was always honest, even when I didn't want to hear it, and she was always there for me, whatever I needed.

But this was different. This time she was flying in from Milwaukee because I had breast cancer. This wasn't a fun road trip or a casual visit. This was serious.

When I spotted her on the sidewalk outside the terminal, something in my chest tightened. Tracy had a way of making everything seem manageable, almost normal—that was until I saw that look in her eye that told me she was worried, which made it impossible for me to pretend I wasn't terrified too.

"So," she said, throwing her carry-on in the trunk of my car, "what's first on the agenda?"

Not "How are you feeling?" or "Are you scared?" Just straight to logistics, to action items, to what needed to be done.

I tried to answer her question about the agenda, but my voice caught. Tracy just pulled me into a hug, right there on the curb despite the honking cars and traffic attendants yelling at us to move the car. "Hey," she said, "we've got this."

We. Not you. *We.*

That's when it hit me. Up until now, it had all been abstract in a way. But having Tracy by my side now meant I could no longer deny that treatment would be starting soon.

The drive home from the airport was a blur of attempted normalcy—catching up on gossip, sharing stories about our kids, planning what needed to be done before surgery. But underneath it all was this new reality that I was about to join the ranks of the patients I'd spent my career treating. And somehow, having my friend here to witness it made it both easier and infinitely more real.

GETTING READY FOR SURGERY

"You're going to need a recliner," Tracy announced on our first full day together. "Trust me on this—you can't lie flat, you can't sleep in your bed, and you'll hate your couch within two days."

That's how we ended up at three different furniture stores, test-driving recliners like they were sports cars. Tracy made me practice getting in and out without using my arms, which earned us some strange looks from salespeople. "You won't be able to push yourself up with your arms," she kept reminding me. "You can't strain your chest muscles. You'll just be an armless torso for the first few weeks."

I was impressed that she knew this. I didn't really see the patients until they were well healed from surgery and had full mobility of their arms. Truthfully, I was unaware of how important guarding the chest wall muscles was. I guess this is what my mother was alluding to when she asked me how I was going to wipe myself because even that motion required stretching the chest wall muscle.

The recliner was just the beginning. My house began to transform into a recovery ward. Prescriptions lined up on the counter. Gauze, surgical bras, and drain management supplies occupied an entire counter in my bathroom. The freezer was filled with premade meals, the pantry was stocked with ramen and boxes of mac and cheese, and the fridge was lined with protein drinks, yogurt, and smoothies for the boys.

I had to undergo several more tests before surgery. Tests that I ordered all the time and provided general descriptions of so patients would know what to expect, even though I had never actually seen any of these tests performed . . . until now.

First up was the breast MRI. Prior to entering the imaging room, I was handed a top, bottom, and a pair of nonslip socks to change into. Everything I wore had to come off; absolutely no metal could be around the MRI since it uses magnetic fields to generate images. Once I was done changing, the technologist placed an IV in my arm for the contrast dye and then led me into the vault.

The machine looked like an elongated donut with a table that slid into the center hole. The tabletop had two openings for the breast to fall through and a face pillow, similar to what you'd find on a massage table. With a little help from the tech, I climbed onto the table and laid on my stomach, positioning my breasts in the openings and resting my face on the pillow. It was not comfortable, and I could easily see why many patients requested Valium to get through this test. Mirrors placed below the face pillow were angled toward the opening of the machine.

"Those mirrors let you see the rest of the room. They're supposed to make it feel less claustrophobic," the tech explained. *Well, they don't*, I thought to myself as the tech positioned my arms above my head and hooked my IV up to the contrast injector. She then placed ear plugs in my ears. "It's going to get really loud in here," she screamed. "Like a bunch of pots and pans banging together. I'll be right outside and can see you through the window. If you have any issues, just wiggle your feet and I'll be right in. You'll be in this position for about thirty minutes. Don't move!"

For the next half hour, I lay awkwardly on my belly with my arms stretched above my head as the table moved me in and out of the machine. But after lying in the machine for what felt like forever, my sternum (aka breastbone) began to hurt, and I couldn't distract myself any longer. I knew I was so close to the end and didn't want to move for fear of messing up the images. So I started counting the seconds . . . one one thousand, two one thousand, three one thousand, four one thousand, five one thousand . . .

It absolutely wasn't working. My chest bone was throbbing at this point. *Keep still, you can do this. Keep still, you don't want to have to come back and do this again*, I repeated to myself inside my head. But the throbbing became more noticeable, and with each passing second, my sternum got more irritated. The throbbing turned into a stabbing-like sensation, and just when I was about to call mercy, the tech slid the table out, disconnected my IV, and said, "All done. I'm going to leave the room and give you some privacy as you get off the table. Your arms are probably asleep, and you may be a little lightheaded, so take you time." As I slowly stood up, I thought to myself, *That test really sucked.*

The PET scan was next on my list, and Tracy decided to accompany me to this test. It wasn't nearly as traumatic as the MRI, but it was a lot of sitting around and waiting. PET stands for positron emission tomography, and it's a scan of tissue activity. Organs that are very active, like the brain and heart, will appear bright. Likewise, tumors also tend to appear bright because they're very active. I had to arrive an hour before the actual scan to receive an injection of radioactive glucose (aka sugar). After I got injected, I sat in a four-by-six-foot room for forty-five minutes to give the glucose time to circulate throughout my entire body. The door to the room was left open, so Tracy pulled up a chair and sat in front of me—still several feet away so she wouldn't be exposed to the small amounts of radioactivity coursing through my veins.

"No talking," the nuclear medicine technician said sternly. "Any movement, including your vocal cords, will concentrate the glucose and give a false read. That means no talking, got it?"

I nodded and sat there, staring at Tracy as she stared back. "Well, this is awkward," I whispered to her.

"Shhhhhhh," she responded seriously. "I was thinking I could talk to you, but I don't want to make you laugh, so just close your eyes and take a nap or something." But I couldn't. This was the scan I was most nervous about. I thought of a patient I'd seen several years ago whose PET scan lit up like a Christmas tree in her abdomen, even though her CT scan was read as unremarkable. Lobular cancer can be difficult to detect on imaging because of its diffuse growth pattern and unusual patterns of spread, like the peritoneum (the lining of the abdomen and pelvis) and gastrointestinal tract. While a PET scan using radioactive glucose wasn't the most sensitive test for my situation, a negative PET scan would reassure me more than the CT I had done a few days prior.

After the waiting period was up, I was led to the PET scanner, which was another donut looking machine. I lay down on my back and tried to think positive, calming thoughts, which didn't work. So I just listened to the sound of the machine as it whirred and felt the table moving my body slowly through the scanner.

When the test was completed, the tech slid me out and asked, "Do you want to see the images?"

I nodded as I sat up. My heart pumped and my pulse raced. This scan would tell me whether I was curable or treatable, the latter indicating metastatic disease that could be controlled but not eradicated. I wanted to know, and I didn't want to know. It's amazing how in a split-second life can go from having endless possibilities to making a bucket list of to-dos before you die. Going forward, I wondered if this would be the thought every time I had any test. I knew the answer was yes, thinking of a beautiful orchid I once received from a patient after I called to tell him that his post-treatment PET scan was all clear. He was so grateful that I called so quickly, as our next appointment was a week away. *Would it ever be possible to get over this fear?*

"It's clear," Tracy said as I entered the control room. I stood next to her, both of us scrolling through the images. "It's clear," she repeated with a sigh of relief, her voice trembling. It was at this moment I realized that she was just as scared and invested in the results of these scans as I was. I then thought of Devina and Wassim too. The speed at which they ordered the tests and got me on the surgery schedule was unreal. The trembling in Tracy's voice reminded me that they were also carrying the anxiety of my diagnosis and overall well-being with them. While we take care of countless breast cancer patients every day, it hits differently when it affects one of your own. I was the one with cancer, but I became ever more aware that we were all in this together.

KEEP CALM AND CARRY ON

Cancer always seems to have a way of messing up schedules. In the office, I've written countless doctor's notes so patients could get a refund or credit on the once-in-a-lifetime trips they've spent years saving up for. But cancer doesn't care about those trips or anything else you have scheduled. It just shows up and expects to become your whole life.

But I couldn't, I *wouldn't*, let it. My kids needed some sense of normalcy to survive this ordeal successfully. I knew that taking a few weeks off from work to recover from the mastectomies would be disorienting enough for them, so I was determined to keep the rest of their lives on track. With the boys in three different schools on three different baseball teams with three different training schedules, I already had a college student helping me get them to where they needed to be. But with me out of the picture, their daily schedule would become a carefully choreographed dance of help from friends, teachers, and coaches.

I was especially determined to maintain my kids' hectic and demanding baseball schedule. Prioritizing baseball while going through cancer treatment may seem like I don't have my priorities straight . . . it *is* youth baseball after all. What's the big deal if they miss a practice or two? But I've instilled in my boys the importance of showing up and fulfilling commitments no matter what is going on in life because there will always be something going on. Leaning into baseball also allowed them to be surrounded by their incredible baseball families, who provided them with endless love and support.

Our new normal wasn't normal at all. It was a constantly shifting landscape of moments when I felt almost like my old self and moments when I wonder if that self would ever return. In those moments, the boys learned to be more independent because they realized they had to. They started doing their own laundry, making their own meals, keeping track of their own schedules. Watching them step up showed me that they were truly capable human beings, if given the opportunity. We were all finding our footing among the chaos. Not because we were trying to be strong but because we had no other choice. We did it because life kept moving forward whether we were ready or not.

A TEAM IN TRANSITION

"I can't do it," Devina said, her voice firm but gentle. "I can't be your lead surgeon. Wassim and I were talking, and he also told me not to do it."

I wasn't surprised when she told me this. I kind of wondered the same thing. While she's one of the best breast surgeons I've ever met, I can't imagine how she would respond if something unforeseen happened in the operating room. I personally wouldn't be able to handle that kind of pressure. I get nervous enough when asked to treat a friend of a friend.

But I was close to all the breast surgeons in the Orlando area and that was a problem. If I wanted to be treated by someone I didn't know, I would have to go outside of the hospital system that I had been affiliated with for the past eight years, which I didn't want to do because I knew and trusted my colleagues.

"Lisa said she'll do it," Devina continued. "Sabrina and Lisa have already coordinated. You need to go to her office tomorrow for the official consult."

I was relieved to hear that Lisa would take control. Lisa was the entire reason the breast cancer program was as reputable as it was. She was a well-regarded breast surgeon who spoke her mind and advocated for her patients. She also had the memory of an elephant, making her a real-life female version of House, the TV show doctor who was able to solve every medical mystery. When I first joined the hospital, she intimidated the heck out of me. She was several years my senior, with an unforgettable head of straight red chin-length hair. She spoke authoritatively and had the respect of all patients. She knew every ounce of data pertaining to breast cancer and practiced like an academician.

Over the years, we became close friends, and I also grew to consider her a mentor—in breast cancer and in life. She, too, was a single mother and had one son. She taught me that honesty was the best policy when talking to my boys about uncomfortable (aka sex) topics. "Connor asked me what sperm was," she recalled one time when we were having lunch. "I told him it was DNA. End of discussion. He got it. There was no giggling, no awkward silence."

While Lisa and I were close, the nature of our relationship was different from my friendship with Devina. Lisa was one step removed, more maternal rather than sisterly, and this step was enough for her to operate objectively. When I got diagnosed, I didn't even realize this was a possibility because Lisa was set to retire on January 28th, and my surgery was scheduled for February 2nd. Ironically, I was supposed to have my mammogram one week earlier than when it happened, but I pushed it off because Devina and I were throwing Lisa's retirement party. We invited 150 of her closest family, friends, and colleagues and arranged for a nine-piece band and fire-eating belly dancer to provide the entertainment. Lisa came dressed like Audrey Hepburn from *Breakfast at Tiffany's*; she was stunning. It was an unforgettable evening and a wonderful way to celebrate her amazing surgical career.

The irony wasn't lost on me. A week ago, I'd been raising a glass to celebrate Lisa's incredible career. Now she was coming back specifically to operate on me. Her party was the last truly good time I had before everything changed.

"We also checked it out with medical staff," Devina informed me. "She's retaining part-time privileges because she has to help me until we can find a suitable replacement, so she's cleared to operate." And just like that, I had a highly qualified breast surgeon that was not also my best friend.

Two days before surgery, Nathan asked me, "Mom, are you going to be able to make your bed after surgery?"

It was such a small thing—making the bed. But it was exactly these small tasks that I wouldn't be able to do. *How was I going to brush my hair? How was I going to wash my hair? How was I going to wash my body?* Each question led me to think of something else I wouldn't be able to do. My mind quickly went into a downward spiral as Nathan stood there waiting for a response. Not wanting to alarm him, I shrugged my shoulders and gave him a kiss goodnight.

Later that evening, I lay awake thinking about Lisa coming out of retirement for me, about Devina stepping aside, about my house filling with medical supplies, and about all the small things that I wouldn't be able to do. It was so overwhelming. *Stop that!* I commanded myself. *You have no reason to feel this way. You know the treatment better than any of your patients and you have tons of support. Lots of women have gotten through breast cancer with much less. Pull it together.*

And then there was the fear I could barely acknowledge: I didn't want to die of this disease. I knew the numbers were on my side but sometimes knowledge doesn't eliminate fear—sometimes knowledge amplifies it. The faces of the patients who failed treatment despite doing everything humanly possible to beat the disease weighed heavily on my mind. Even though I knew they were the minority, it was impossible not to see myself in those who failed.

THE BOOBIE FAIRY VISITS

"We're stopping by in a few minutes," Andrea and Alicja told me in unison over the phone. "We want to say goodbye to your boobs."

I laughed as they hung up the phone. I was so fortunate to have made wonderful adult friends when I moved to Orlando. An incredible job opportunity brought me to Florida, but it was a little daunting to relocate to a new city where my family and I knew no one. I decided the best way for the kids to make friends would be to register them for soccer because it seemed like everyone played soccer in Florida. At the age of seven, James was randomly assigned to a team that was coached by Andrea's husband, Kevin. Her oldest son, Alden, and Alicja's only son, Ethan, were on the team and the three of them became fast friends.

Alicja and I struck up an instant friendship as we cheered from the sidelines. She was a blonde-haired, blue-eyed Polish beauty who appeared calm and collected until an unfair call was made against *her* Ethan. Then the momma bear would come out, and she would give the ref a piece of her mind. She had no problem yelling at others in her sharp, Eastern European accent that easily instilled fear in those around her. It was entertaining to watch and sometimes cringeworthy when she made a comment that went too far. I was actually amazed that she never got ejected from a game.

Andrea took me a little longer to befriend because she was never around when James first joined the team. I initially thought Kevin was a single father, then soon learned that she wasn't at the games because she was at home taking care of their newborn baby. Eventually Andrea started showing up and we instantly hit it off. Like Alicja, she also had blonde hair and blue eyes, but she was from Minnesota. She was a former D1 collegiate volleyball player who single-handedly renovated her home while working as a full-time occupational therapist for the school district.

She and Kevin are two of the kindest people I have ever met, always offering to help me with my boys even though they had three children themselves. They are also an amazingly fun couple and even more incredible as friends, looking out for me and the boys in every respect.

Over a short period of time, Alicja, Andrea, Kevin, and I formed a tight bond and became each other's extended family. We celebrated holidays and traveled on vacations together. As the boys got older, they transitioned from soccer to baseball and we turned every tournament into a mini-vacation. We always managed to have a good time together, even if that good time was sitting in the car for two hours waiting for a lightning delay to pass.

The night before my mastectomies, Tracy and I were in my kitchen doing last-minute preparations when the garage door creaked open, followed by a strange high-pitched voice—something between Mrs. Doubtfire and a fairy godmother.

In walked Andrea, all six feet of her, wearing a fluorescent pink wig, pink heart-shaped sunglasses, a tight black shirt with two pink balloons popping out from her chest and a pink sequin mini-skirt, complete with angel wings and a bubble wand. She pranced around me in circles, blowing bubbles everywhere.

"Hello . . . hello! Well hello there! I'm the boobie fairy! I'm here to say goodbye to your boobies!" she exclaimed, doing her best not to laugh.

I started laughing, really laughing, for what felt like the first time since my diagnosis.

She blew bubbles at my breasts and tapped each one with her wand and waved them goodbye. "So long, girls, so long" she sang.

"Thank you for your service, but it is time for you to go." She then chest bumped me and took a bow.

Tracy, Alicja, Andrea, and I all stood there in the kitchen laughing uncontrollably.

"It's so kind of you to come," I giggled as I squeezed the pink balloon breasts busting out of her shirt.

"Let's not forget the gifts!" Andrea exclaimed. Alicja stepped forward with several gift bags, each containing something I would need during my recovery. There was a plush pink robe, a button-down shirt with drain holders in the side, a blanket, and a black string bracelet with "F.U. CANCER" written in Morse Code.

"We will be by tomorrow when you get home," Alicja added. "I will bring chicken soup. Do you need anything else?"

I shook my head. I was so grateful for my friends and for being able to find humor, even in the darkest of moments. I looked at Andrea, who began to blow bubbles again, and giggled.

She looked amazing and ridiculous at the same time.

It was perfect. It was just what I needed twelve hours before going into surgery.

SAYING GOODBYE

After the Boobie Fairy and Alicja left, I had to say goodbye to my dogs Charlie and Layla. I initially planned to keep all three at home with me during my recovery, but Tracy and Devina nixed that idea quickly.

"Sue, you are going to have drains coming out of your chest wall for at least one to two weeks," Devina said sternly. "You will have FOUR open holes, FOUR potential areas that bacteria and viruses can enter your body."

"You don't want your reconstruction to fail," Tracy chimed in. "We all know how hard it is to recover from this kind of infection.

These dogs are like your shadow. They follow your every step as soon as you enter the house."

"You know," Devina added, "some plastic surgeons tell their patients to send their pets away during this time. Sabrina didn't, but that doesn't mean you shouldn't take this seriously."

With both of them scolding me, I arranged for friends to take Layla and Charlie for the next two weeks. But Zeus had to stay with me because he needed my large fenced-in backyard to run around. Despite his shady beginnings of being purchased in the parking lot of a Walgreens, he grew into an impressively muscular dog with an intimidating presence at one hundred and eighty-five pounds. His sheer size and unpredictable behavior toward unfamiliar humans and dogs made walking him on a leash impossible. When he was younger and about thirty pounds lighter, I was able to take him on evening strolls. But that abruptly came to an end the day he decided to charge full speed, while growling and baring his teeth, at a neighbor who also happened to be a highly successful personal injury attorney. I held on to his leash as best I could, screaming "Stop!" But my one-hundred-and-fifty-pound frame did nothing to slow him down. Thankfully, he lost interest when he got within fifteen feet of the neighbor, who stood still with a look of *Bring it on*. After that day, I thought it was best from a safety and liability perspective to never walk Zeus again.

I gave Layla and Charlie a big hug as I said goodbye. I looked them in the eyes and thought, *The next time I see you, I won't have breasts*. My normal life, partly defined by my three dogs, was being deconstructed. I knew the dogs would be back, but their departure meant I was one step closer to go time.

Tracy slept in the master with me that last night. She didn't make a big deal about it, just set up camp in my room like we were having a sleepover. Her presence was both comforting and terrifying—comforting because she was there and terrifying because she felt she needed to be.

My support system was now fully activated. My colleagues were now my care team. My friends were now my lifelines. My kids were now my protectors. And I was trying to hold it all together while simultaneously falling apart.

In all my years of practicing medicine, I never fully understood the emotional weight of the night before surgery. I would always tell my patients to get a good night's rest and to stay positive. That night, I made a mental note to not tell them this anymore as I lay wide awake. I also remembered my last conversation with Lisa, who stopped by to check on me two days before surgery.

"You're going to have to find someone to wipe your butt," she told me matter-of-factly.

"Oh my God, how did my mom get a hold of you?" I asked.

"You can't move any of this," she gestured to my upper body ignoring my question. "How are you going to reach back there?"

I remembered thinking, *I'll find a way. No one is wiping my butt.* But with surgery now hours away, I was about to lose my independence in the most basic ways. As I lay there in the dark, listening to Zeus snore away, I realized something: I've spent my whole life doing everything by myself. Maybe this is my body telling me it's time to stop that and it's time to start letting people in. While I considered my independence to be one of my greatest strengths, perhaps it was also one of my greatest weaknesses because it prevented me from fully trusting and relying on others. And as I tried to figure out the *why* to my diagnosis, maybe this was the universe's way of telling me that we all need to depend on each other to survive and, more importantly, to thrive.

I didn't sleep much that night, so when the alarm went off at 4:30 A.M., I jumped out of bed and turned on the shower. As I waited for the water to heat up, I took off my clothes and stood in front of the bathroom mirror. *Well, girls,* I thought, *this is it. Today, we say goodbye.* Breastfeeding three babies had definitely taken its toll on them. They were perky for my age, but I could tell that if they were given another ten years, they would look like pancakes. Guess it's better to go out now while they are still in their prime, rather than watch them wither away.

After I took a shower, Tracy knocked on the bathroom door. "Are you ready?" she asked. "You have to check in at the registration desk at 5:30."

"Let me just say goodbye to the boys," I said quietly.

Nathan's room was the closest. When I entered his room, he was wrapped up in his blanket like a burrito with only his head and feet sticking out. He was typically an early riser and opened his eyes when I came in. "Can you come and lay down with me, Mommy?" he asked so innocently. I couldn't remember the last time he called me mommy. At eleven years old, he was always testing the boundaries of respect and would use "Ma," "bruh," and occasionally "Hey, you" to get my attention. I lay down next to him for a few minutes and hugged him tightly. I told him I loved him and gave him a kiss on the cheek. Before I left his room, I tickled his feet to make him giggle and then tucked them tightly in the blanket.

I wandered up the stairs to Sam's room next. Sam loved to sleep in subarctic temperatures, so a blast of cold air hit my face and goosebumps formed on my arms and legs as I entered. I sat at the foot of his bed and watched him sleep, which I did often when he was little. As a baby, he loved to sleep with his arms above his head no matter how tightly I bundled him up with his arms tight by his side. Now as I sat there watching him as a teenager, I was amused to notice that he still slept with his arms above his head.

I got up, gave him a kiss on his forehead, whispered I loved him, and closed his door on my way down the stairs.

One more goodbye, I thought to myself as I walked over to James's room. Zeus had made his way to James's bed while I was in the shower, leaving his door ajar. James' king bed was pushed to the corner and he always slept diagonally with his head in the corner. *You always make things difficult for me, don't you?* I thought as I got on all fours and crawled very slowly to the corner of the bed. I was about to give him a kiss on his forehead when his eyes opened. He sat up quickly, headbutting me in the chin, and screamed, "What the f—"

I rubbed my chin and said, "I just wanted to tell you I love you and say goodbye. Tracy is taking me to the hospital now."

"What time is it?" he asked.

"Five," I responded as I gave him a kiss on the cheek.

"Good, I can get another hour of sleep," he sighed as he pulled the covers over his head.

As I made my way out of his room, I was hurt that he didn't say something more heartfelt. But just as I was about to close his door, I heard him call out, "Mom . . ."

"Yes, buddy?"

"I love you."

"Love you too. I'll see you tonight."

Tracy was waiting for me in the car. It was a pretty quiet ride to the hospital. Neither of us wanted to talk. Walking into the hospital as a patient instead of a doctor was like stepping into a parallel universe—everything familiar yet completely foreign. Everything smelled the same and looked the same, but nothing felt the same. After I completed patient registration, I was taken to a pre-op holding room where the TV was already on. Q, Devina's husband, was on the morning news—a strange moment of normalcy in what was about to be the least normal day of my life. I watched him report live from outside someone's house. I couldn't hear what he was saying, but it didn't matter because I was thinking how for everyone else, this was just another Friday.

Once I changed into the hospital gown and climbed onto the bed, the enormity of what was about to happen hit me like a ton of bricks. Tracy sat at my bedside, but I couldn't bear to look at her. I knew she was getting teary-eyed. Then Devina walked in. Despite the huge smile on her face, her body language was so stiff and unnatural that I knew she was nervous about the day ahead. Her level of concern was palpable, and I couldn't hold back any longer. My eyes began to water and my nose started to run. Then Tracy gulped as she tried to choke back a sob.

At that moment, the anesthesiologist entered. She was seven months pregnant and totally unaware of what she was walking into. She leaned on the side of my bed and looked at me. When our eyes made contact, tears started streaming down my cheeks. I didn't even know her, but something about her presence—about her creating life while I was fighting to preserve mine—broke something loose in me.

"Oh no, don't cry" she said as she handed me a box of tissues. "It'll be okay. I just wanted to introduce myself. I'm Jasmine, and I'll be your anesthesiologist. Can you tell me what procedure we are performing today?"

I took a few deep breaths and was able to control my emotions long enough to answer her questions. I looked over at Devina and Tracy, who both had bloodshot eyes from crying quietly in the corner. Outside the room, Lisa was talking to the nurses. Hearing her give orders to the staff made the reality of what was about to happen undeniable. There was no stopping this train.

Lisa peeked her head through the curtain. "Are you hanging in there?" she asked as she entered the room and patted the back of my hands. I started crying again. But this time it was a full-on ugly cry, a first for me since this entire journey began. I kept thinking, *Why me*, but I knew better than to ask a question that no one in the room could answer. I looked Lisa in the eyes and could see a glimmer of tears. But she was able to maintain her composure. "I knew you didn't want me to retire, but don't you think you've gone a little too far this time?" she joked.

I chuckled. I always appreciated her wit and ability to crack a wiseass comment when I least expected it. And while I knew she was joking, I felt bad for dragging her back into the OR. She had worked so hard for so many years and deserved a peaceful retirement with no more early morning surgeries and long OR days. But here she was, "officially" retired on Monday yet back in the operating room on Friday to help a friend in need.

The plastic surgery team then entered the room. "Okay, let's get you up," Sabrina instructed as her PA, Sophie, lowered the guard rail and helped me out of the bed and onto my feet. "I need to mark you before we go to surgery." Everyone had seen my breasts at this point, so I just dropped my gown to my waist. Sabrina took out her marker, held the cap between her teeth, and started drawing lines all over my chest. She then drew a semicircle just outside my left areola to indicate where she intended to lift the nipple. As she scooted back in the stool to make sure her markings were symmetrical, I developed a whole new appreciation for her ability to remain professionally detached. Despite the fact that I stood there sniffling away, she maintained total control of her emotions as she visualized what she was going to do.

"Okay, everything looks great!" she exclaimed as she capped the marker and helped me back into bed. "You are going to look fabulous, darling."

Just then, another head peaked through the curtain. "Hello?" Anu whispered softly. "I hope you don't mind, but I heard what was going on and wanted to be here for you." She gave me a hug and then took my hands in hers. She mouthed the words, *It's going to be okay*, as her eyes started to moisten with tears. I nodded back, doing my best to believe her.

I first met Anu when she stopped by my office to introduce herself as a new breast surgeon in town. She was warm and friendly while simultaneously exuding a "Don't screw me or I will take you down" attitude, despite being only five foot one. She was also the mother of three boys, the oldest who made the local news when he decided he wanted out of her womb during Hurricane Sandy (aka the Storm of the Century). I always got a good laugh when she tells the story of going into labor while all lower Manhattan had no electricity; she had to be carried down forty flights of stairs by four firefighters because she was ginormous (her word, not mine).

I looked at the clock, it was almost time to go. I looked around the room. Typically, only two people were allowed to accompany the patient in pre-op holding, but it was standing room only in mine as everyone crowded around my bedside.

Jasmine re-entered the room with her nurse anesthetist, Hector. "Holy moly," he exclaimed. "Well, this is the place to be! All the pretty ladies are here, and we have the drugs. Are you ready to get this party started?" he asked with a huge smile on his face. And just like that, the somber mood was broken.

"Time for the ESP block," Jasmine interrupted. "I need you to swing your legs around the bed and lean on this table." Devina moved in front of me to hold my hands, Lisa left the room to change into her scrubs, and Tracy moved to stand by Anu and Sabrina in the corner of the room.

"I'm going to inject the long-acting numbing medication Exparel into your back muscle, near your spine, to block the chest wall nerves from sending pain signals to your brain. These nerves will be really irritated the first few days after the mastectomies. The block lasts two to three days and minimizes the need for narcotics." *Great,* I thought to myself, but an injection into the deep back muscles sounded *really freaking* painful.

"But before the block," Jasmine continued, "I'm going to give you Versed. Do you want to say anything to anyone before the Versed? Because once you get it, you won't remember a thing."

I found it hard to believe that I wouldn't remember anything despite being awake, but I took her at her word. I looked around the room one more time. "Let's do this."

I watched Jasmine inject Versed into my IV.

And she was right. I have absolutely no recollection of what happened for the next ten hours.

THE LONG WAKE-UP

Recovery was a blur of familiar faces in unfamiliar contexts. Devina and Tracy were there, their voices floating in and out of my consciousness. I remember insisting I was ready to go home and someone—probably Tracy—saying, "You were under anesthesia for almost eight hours. You're not ready to go home."

They were right, of course. When I finally made it back to my house, twelve hours after leaving, everything was spinning as I sat back in my recliner. My vision was also off—a side effect of the anesthesia no one had warned me about, or maybe they had? My near vision was so bad I had to hold my phone three feet in front of my face to read the barrage of incoming texts from my family and friends.

I also had an insatiable craving for salt, so I kept asking for Takis and Cheetos, which my kids gladly fed me as they took turns throwing pieces in my gaping mouth like it was a carnival game. I dozed off in the recliner, and when I awoke, Andrea, Alicja, Devina, and Tracy were sitting in my bed watching TV.

"Chicken soup?" Alicja asked. I nodded, and within seconds she was at my side spoon-feeding me soup so I could rest my arms.

I dozed off again, and the next time I woke up, my bedroom was dark, but the light from the hallway was still on. An unopened box of saltines and six empty bags of chips (snack size, not party) sat on the table next to me. I could hear Zeus snoring on the bed, and when I looked over at him, I saw Devina curled up next to him. I had to go to the bathroom but didn't want to wake her because I knew how stressful the day was for her. I had minimal discomfort, so I thought, *How hard can it be to go to the bathroom by myself?* Thank God, I just had to pee because I still hadn't figured out how I would wipe by backside.

My fingers felt the side of the recliner for the buttons that would raise my back up. Once I was in the seated position, I still struggled because my legs felt so weak. I started to rock my torso back and forth to build enough momentum to propel me forward. But my butt sank so far into the seat that rocking didn't do anything.

"Devina?" I whispered. No response.

"Devina?" I spoke a little louder. No response.

I really needed to pee, so I put my arms down on the armrests and pushed up. A searing pain shot through my anterior chest wall, *Oh crap . . . I hope I didn't just rip something.* But it felt like a victory because I was up on my own two feet. I slowly shuffled towards the bathroom, putting my hands on the nearby wall to steady myself. I stopped with each step because I felt so light-headed. *Don't fall. Don't fall. That would really piss Devina and Tracy off.* It took five minutes to make my way to the toilet, a route that only took five seconds twenty-four hours before. When I finally sat down, it felt like the best pee of my life but then I realized, *Oh crap, I have to stand up again.* It was my first real test of independence, and it was humbling. Everything hurt and the simplest tasks became monumental challenges.

In all my years of treating breast cancer patients, I'd explained the basic principles of the surgery. I'd gone over the recovery process, discussed pain management, and warned about movement restrictions. But no amount of medical knowledge could have prepared me for the sheer physical reality of it—the way every breath reminded me of what had been done to my body.

That first night, drifting in and out of consciousness in my recliner, I realized this was just the beginning. The surgery might be over, but the real work of recovery was just starting. And despite all my professional experience, I was just as vulnerable and uncertain as any other patient facing this journey. And somehow, this realization was simultaneously terrifying and liberating.

Chapter Four

MORE BAD NEWS

My house looked like someone had just died.

Between the casseroles and the flowers, it reminded me of what homes look like after a family member passes. Every surface held either a bouquet or a covered dish, creating this surreal landscape of sympathy and support. The scent of lilies, roses, and tulips mixed with the aroma of what seemed like every comfort food known to mankind.

I was still foggy from anesthesia, but the sight was overwhelming. Flowers had been trickling in since the diagnosis, and now some arrangements were clearly on their way out, drooping and shedding petals while fresh ones stood proudly beside them. It was like watching time-lapse photography of hope and decay, all at once.

I'd never been much of a flower person. Too practical, maybe—the daughter of immigrants who wore clothes from the 1970s and saved every penny for their children's education. Sixty dollars for something that would die in seven to ten days seemed wasteful. But standing there, I understood for the first time why people send them. They were a visible reminder that people cared, that they were thinking of you, that they wanted to do something—anything—to help.

Still, the sheer volume was overwhelming. Every day, I'd wake up confused, trying to orient myself in my transformed house. The cavalry had arrived in full force, bearing petals and pasta, and I had no idea how to handle it.

The recliner became my new world. Sleeping in a bed was impossible with the four drains coming out of my chest wall. As uncomfortable as they were, they were absolutely necessary for the first few weeks after surgery to prevent fluid from building up inside my body. My bedroom was transformed into a medical command center, with supplies organized on every surface and a rotation of caretakers always within earshot.

I'd tried to prepare myself for the pain, but nothing really prepares you for the constant awareness of your chest, the way every movement requires careful calculation. Simple tasks became elaborate puzzles: how to reach for water, how to stand up, how to exist in a body that suddenly felt like a stranger.

The meal train, something that I initially said no to thinking that my kids could UberEats all their meals, became a blessing I never knew I needed. Despite my objection, Marie, the mother hen of my department, was now mothering me at home and insisted on organizing one. Once the food started arriving, I realized that while the actual food helped nourish my family's bodies, the care and thought that went into preparing or ordering the meals helped nourish my family's spirit.

Our first meal was from a father-like coworker, a wonderful gentleman who really enjoyed Southern food and made a great Santa Claus during the holidays. He sent both fried and rotisserie chicken, apparently hedging his bets knowing how I liked to eat clean. There was also potato salad, coleslaw, macaroni salad, and two types of pie. I looked at this feast of comfort food, deeply touched but also thinking, *I don't eat any of this.* My kids, on the other hand, were delighted to finally have some "good stuff" at the house and devoured it all in one sitting.

Every day brought new visitors, new food, new care packages. The generosity was overwhelming, but so was the social obligation it created. I was exhausted, in pain, and somehow still feeling guilty about not being a better host to the people stopping by to visit. Thankfully, Tracy ran interference in the early days after surgery. "You don't have to entertain people," she kept reminding me. "They're here to help."

She also kept the home organized. "We should probably throw some of these away," she suggested, referring to the arrangements I received just after my diagnosis. "The kids need space to do their homework, and I'm sure flowers all over the place are making it difficult for them to concentrate. And you hate clutter, so cleaning up a little will make it easier for you all to relax in your space."

I nodded, watching her throw out two bouquets of wilted flowers and wash out the vases. *Living. Right.* That's what all this was about, wasn't it? The flowers, the food, the friends camping out on my couch—it wasn't about dying. It was about living through this—even if right now, my house looked like a place where hope came to wilt.

THE NIPPLE CHRONICLES

Recovery comes with its own vocabulary. Words like "drain output" and "cc measurement" become part of daily conversation. My medical knowledge didn't make the reality of stripping drains any less unpleasant nor did it make the sight of tubes emerging from my body any less alien.

Tracy managed it all the first few days after surgery with characteristic efficiency. "Fifteen cc's on the right, twenty on the left," she'd note, keeping meticulous records. Meanwhile, I tried not to think about how many times I'd told patients this part would be "a bit uncomfortable." Uncomfortable didn't begin to cover it. You don't feel human when you have four drains coming out of your body.

Three days after surgery, Tracy had to get back to her life. Q arrived at my house to drive her to the airport, and I was forbidden from going with them. "If it's a bumpy car ride, you'll be really uncomfortable," Tracy told me. "I don't like long goodbyes anyway. I'm sure we will see each other soon enough." She gave me a quick hug and got in the car. And just like that, Tracy and Q drove away as I stood in the driveway unable to wave goodbye.

With Tracy gone, Devina now became my primary caregiver. She stopped by after she finished her last surgery of the day to assume drain-stripping duties.

"Have you bathed since the surgery?" she asked as she poured the fluid from the drain bulb into the measuring cup.

"Nope."

"You should get in the bath tonight, waist down." She said it like a suggestion, but it really was more of a command.

"I showered the morning of surgery," I replied. "I think I can get away with a few more days of just wiping down with bath wipes. Besides, it's just me and you, so I don't care if I smell." The truth? It was hard enough to stand up. I didn't know how I was going to possibly lower myself into a bathtub.

"You are acting like a child. I'm going to start the bath, and you are going to get in. End of discussion." When the tub had about six inches of water, she shut off the faucet and said, "Okay, let's get you in."

I gave her an odd look. It's one thing for her to see me naked from waist up, but waist down?

"I can do this myself," I said as I pointed her to the door.

"No, you can't. Let me help you take off your pants and underwear. There's no way you can get in this bath by yourself. This is exactly why I'm here. Let me help you," she insisted.

I continued to refuse, pointing her to the door. I knew that as a doctor she had seen it all before, but she had never seen all of me before . . . and it just felt awkward.

"Sue, what is the big deal?" she finally asked in frustration. "I've already seen you down there. I was the one who put in your catheter at the time of the surgery." And with that, I let her help me. Knowing that she already saw that part of me, even though I was out cold, suddenly made it okay.

She helped me slowly ease down into the tub and I had to admit that the warm water felt so comforting against my skin. Once I completed bathing, she slid her arms under my armpits and lifted me gently up. As I dried off, I thanked her for her help because there was no way I could have done that myself.

After I got dressed, Devina suggested that we look at the reconstruction, and I agreed.

"I know you will like how it turned out," she said confidently as she unwrapped the bandages. "The first set that Sabrina put in during the surgery was way too big. I told her that you would kill me if we left those in." She giggled. "But when she put these implants in, we all thought you looked perfect. What do you think?"

She took a step back and started rerolling the long bandage back up. The first time I looked in the mirror, panic hit hard. As I stared down at my new breasts, I did a double take at my left nipple. "Is my nipple black?!" I asked Devina.

She stopped what she was doing, took a look, and paused just a moment too long. "Huh."

"Oh, is that supposed to be like, 'Huh, interesting' or 'Huh, this is really bad'?"

She didn't respond. She reached for her cell phone. "Can I take a quick pic? I want to see what Sabrina thinks."

Great, I thought, *my nipple is dying.* As we waited for Sabrina to text back, I thought about one patient I had whose nipples didn't survive the reconstruction. "It was the strangest thing, Doc," the patient recounted. "The nipples turned black, and after a few days, they just fell off."

As I mentally prepared myself for Sabrina to declare my nipple dead, I starting running through which tattoo artist I would visit to get 3D nipple tattoos.

Devina's phone dinged. I tried to peek over her shoulder to read the text, but she intentionally blocked my view. "You're good," Devina informed me with a smile. "Sabrina said put some Silvadene on it. The top layer of the nipple is just sloughing off. Give it a few days, and it'll be fine."

I was so relieved, but that moment of panic—of watching my friend and colleague try to maintain professional calm while documenting my potentially dying nipple—crystallized the strange space I was inhabiting of late.

INITIAL STEPS FORWARD

"When can I get my Lupron?" I texted Wassim. I was only a few days post-op, but I wanted to start the next part of my treatment yesterday. The MammaPrint test that he ordered on my biopsy specimen showed I had low risk disease so endocrine therapy would be all that I needed. No chemo thank goodness! But knowing that my disease was ER positive, meaning that I had cancer that grew in the presence of estrogen, and knowing that my ovaries were still obliviously pumping out estrogen gave me so much anxiety. Surgery did an excellent job of putting out the fire, but embers were very likely still present. The thought of estrogen circulating through my premenopausal body left me with images of gasoline being sprayed over the embers, leaving the possibility for another fire to erupt at any moment.

"You just had surgery. Let's wait a few weeks," he replied. I knew the reason for waiting was to give patients time to recover from the mastectomies. I would always tell patients, "Get over one set of side effects before you start another, especially when the next treatment will bring a whole other set of side effects."

"I understand the reason for waiting, but I want to start hormonal suppression now. I'm well aware of what the side effects are, and I'm ready for them. I can't sit one more day knowing that my ovaries are pumping out estrogen like nothing ever happened. PLEASE, SHUT THEM DOWN NOW." I pleaded.

"Okay. I'll put the order in. Go to the infusion center today when you have time."

While the physical limitations of surgery were impossible to ignore, I was ready for this next step. I was well versed on the menopausal symptoms that Lupron was notorious for. But menopause is a natural process that all women will go through as they age . . . how hard could it be?

THE DAY EVERYTHING CHANGED (AGAIN)

It was a Wednesday, five days after the mastectomies, and the results from my surgery were still not back. In the real world, this timeline would be normal. But I knew the pathologist reading my case, and I was also aware that Wassim, Devina, and Lisa had requested it be read quickly. So where was my full report?

Finally, at noon, I called Wassim. "Where the heck is my path? What's going on here?"

"Let me call them again," Wassim said with an undertone of *Don't call me again about this. I'll call you once it's back.*

The delay prepared me for results that weren't good. If the pathology was straightforward, it would have gone through a double check, and the results would have been released. If the pathology is a little bit more complex, then it typically gets reviewed internally several more times before the results are officially signed off for the oncologist and patient to discuss.

Julie, my practice manager, was working from my house that day to keep me company. I'd met her my first day on the job, and she was someone whose bad side you did not want to get on. She managed our clinic schedules, call schedules, and vacation schedules; dealt with upper administration on our behalf; and made sure we were up to date on our licenses and practice privileges. She was on top of issues before they even arose and prevented our group from falling into utter disarray. She stayed with us as we grew from seven providers to more than thirty, which meant that she loved a good challenge and was loyal to our group.

After a few hours, Devina showed up. "Did you hear from Wassim yet?" she asked as soon as she came in.

"Nope."

At this point, Julie started cleaning my countertops and reorganizing my pantry. "Just trying to keep busy," she told me. I knew better, though. She was getting nervous as we waited for the results. Whenever she gets nervous, she starts cleaning. She did it when she came to visit me in my office, and she was now doing it in my home.

Just then, Lisa called. "I have the pathology back." I put the phone on speaker, and Devina, Julie, and I huddled around it.

"There was a lot of disease in your breast Sue, they stopped counting after ten tumors. Total extent of invasive disease was measured at eleven centimeters . . ." Her voice trailed off.

"Okay . . . what about the lymph nodes?" I asked nervously. With that much disease in the breast and having a lobular histology, I had prepared myself for the worst.

"Negative," she reported. "Five were removed, and they are all negative."

"So no chemo right?" Devina asked. "The MammaPrint was low risk, so that means no chemo . . ."

"Just one thing, Sue," Lisa interrupted. "There was extensive pleomorphic lobular carcinoma in situ, and this extended to the anterior, superior, and inferior margins. So technically you have positive margins."

I felt like I'd just been punched in the gut. I totally didn't see that one coming. Pleomorphic lobular carcinoma in situ is treated like ductal carcinoma in situ (aka Stage 0 breast cancer), meaning my surgery left behind residual disease. The margins were positive, meaning I had a high risk of local recurrence if I didn't do anything else. So I needed more surgery or I needed radiation.

When I headed into surgery, I was not anticipating an issue with margins. While I had multiple tumors in the breast, radiation recommendations are typically based on the size of the largest tumor, which was three point six centimeters and not big enough to need radiation. And even though I had a lymph node involved, after a thorough review, we all agreed it was a lymph node in axillary breast tissue, and not a true axillary lymph node. So my expectation was no radiation if my axillary lymph nodes at the time of surgery were negative.

"We can try to take you back to surgery to find those margins," Lisa thought aloud. "But it will be a struggle to know if the additional tissue we take is from the area of concern or some other area."

"On top of that, your flaps are really thin," Devina added. "If we try to go after those margins, I'm not sure how much tissue we can get, and the flaps can be compromised. Your reconstruction might not end up looking as good."

I knew what both of them were getting at. They could take me back to surgery if I wanted, but they really didn't advise it. If this were any other patient, re-excision would not have even been discussed due to how many positive margins there were. They would have just sent this patient straight to me for radiation. But this wasn't any other patient, it was me . . . and I was a radiation oncologist that did not want radiation.

While undergoing mastectomies was traumatic, knowing that the reconstruction would preserve the way I looked played an integral part in my healing process and ability to move on with life after cancer. I was still recovering, but my implants looked excellent, minus the black nipple that I was assured was just temporary. The addition of radiation, which is only recommended for patients at high risk of local recurrence, could cause the implant to look firmer, smaller, and lifted. Quite honestly, what I did for a living could really screw up the reconstruction.

I always told patients in my situation that the goal of a radiation oncologist and the goal of a plastic surgeon are on opposite sides of the scale. Obviously, oncologic outcome is always more important than cosmetic outcome but knowing first-hand how damaging treatment could be and the psychological effects it had on my patients terrified me. My desire to put this all behind me quickly would be virtually impossible if I had to see a cosmetically deformed breast every day for the rest of my life, with the biggest irony being that the deformation was caused by something I've built my career on.

As a physician, I was always so objective and even matter of fact when discussing radiation-related complications in this setting. In my doctor mind, who cares about what the implant looks like in a few years? If we can't get control of this disease now, it will kill you, and you won't be around to worry about the implant. I truly didn't understand how some patients were more worried about how the implant looked than controlling the cancer. And now here I was, being that patient I would have judged so harshly a few weeks ago for trying to get out of a treatment that the medical side of me knew I needed.

"Let's call Tracy and ask her," I said calmly as I picked up my phone. She was with a patient at the time but was anxiously awaiting my call, so she stepped out of the room to answer the phone. I read her the report, and without hesitation, she said, "You need radiation."

I then called my partner, Wes. We both started working for the group at the same time. His life before medicine made him an interesting person to talk to. He quite literally joined the circus after he graduated from Florida State University, which apparently had a circus program. (Who knew?) Then, he joined a band and traveled around performing for a few years. Eventually, he found his way to medicine, which I was very thankful for because I always used him as a sounding board when I had a difficult case. He was data driven and could quote numbers from any study that was brought up.

"Hey, I just texted you a path report. Do you think this patient needs radiation?" I asked him.

After a few minutes of silence, he said, "This is you, isn't it?"

"Yes," I responded quietly.

"I'm sorry, Sue. I think you know my answer."

I was determined to find someone that thought otherwise. I proceeded to call a co-resident that trained with me at Northwestern, a former attending that I trained under, as well as the head of breast radiation oncology at UPenn. Tracy consulted her partners at the Medical College of Wisconsin as well. Everyone came back with the same recommendation.

In a final effort to get out of radiation, I called Na'im, the head of the pathology department who specialized in breast cancer. In our limited interactions, his high level of intelligence was always obvious. He was the ultimate medical detective, examining microscopic clues to solve what was going on with the patient. All medical decisions are based off his interpretation of what he sees. Often at tumor board, he would show pictures of his findings, while using words like nuclear pleomorphism, tubular differentiation, and proliferation index to describe his thought process. Meanwhile, I would sit there appreciating the artistic nature of his slides while sometimes getting befuddled in his medical terminology. I trusted him implicitly.

"Hey," I said cheerfully. "I'm really sorry to bother you, but can I ask you a question about my pathology?"

"Of course, Sue. Whatever you need," he responded with a typical kindness in his voice that I was so used to hearing from him.

"What's the deal with the margins? And is the LCIS really pleomorphic? And my understanding is that the disease is one big tumor surrounded by a bunch of satellite nodules, so why was the size of the invasive component reported at eleven centimeters?" I spat out a few more questions than I planned, but I figured if I had him on the phone, I might as well get answers for everything I was wondering.

He took his time explaining to me what he saw underneath the microscope and his rationale for reporting what he did. I didn't question anything he told me. I knew I didn't really need to call him, but I was grasping for straws at this point. He shared his findings and then as we ended our conversation, he said, "Sue, I thought about reaching out to you sooner on multiple occasions, but I didn't want to be too intrusive. I want you to know that you have been on all of our minds. I'm so sorry that you are going through this, and I'm so sorry I couldn't give you better news." There was an undeniable tone of sadness in his voice. It wasn't a sadness that came from having to tell me that I had cancer; it was a sadness that came from having to tell me that I had extensive cancer, and he knew exactly what it meant.

When I hung up the phone, I accepted the fact that radiation was in my future.

"Well," I said as I went to the freezer looking for some Jeni's Gooey Butter Cake ice cream to comfort me. "At least I don't need chemo."

I grabbed two spoons and sat down on the couch next to Devina. I waved a spoon at Julie, who moved on to sweeping the floors. "Let me just finish the floors first," she said.

Devina, who was a bodybuilder in her spare time and ate *extremely* clean, watched me as I dug into the ice cream. My phone rang again, and she got up to answer it. "Hey, Wassim. You're on speaker. We just talked to Lisa, and she told us the path. We know Sue needs radiation."

"She also needs chemo," he said unexpectedly. I stopped eating ice cream, and Julie stopped sweeping the floors.

"What do you mean?" I questioned. "My genomic testing showed low-risk disease."

"I know, but you are clinically high risk," he explained. "You are premenopausal, you had a positive lymph node, and you had extensive disease."

"But genomic testing was low risk," I interjected.

"But you are clinically high risk." He repeated the statement slowly and authoritatively.

I didn't say anything. I couldn't say anything. Just an hour ago, I thought the mastectomies would be the worst of it. I needed to get back to work. I needed to get back to my kids. I needed to get back to my life. I didn't have time for this. Now, I was being told I needed chemo in addition to radiation, which would set me back another four months.

"You had so many tumors in the breast. I'm going to run genomic testing on some of the other larger tumors. Regardless of the results, though, my recommendation is chemotherapy." Wassim wasn't talking to me as a friend; he was talking to me as my doctor.

The three of us stood in my kitchen silently. That was not at all what we were expecting to hear.

Julie resumed cleaning. I resumed eating ice cream. Devina sat down next to me, grabbed the second spoon and started eating ice cream too. I started crying when she did this because I couldn't remember the last time I'd seen her eat ice cream. Then Devina started crying. Julie kept cleaning, moving from room to room like she could somehow restore order to my life by organizing my house. The house smelled like Pine-Sol and despair.

That's the thing about bad news in medicine—it rarely comes all at once. It creeps in slowly, building detail by detail into something bigger and scarier than you initially imagined. I thought the surgery was the hard part. Now I was realizing it was just the beginning.

The ice cream helped a little. Julie's cleaning helped in its own way. Devina's presence helped most of all. But nothing could completely ease the weight of knowing that this journey was going to be longer and harder than I expected. The path forward was suddenly much less clear and much more daunting.

And somewhere in the back of my mind, I could hear myself saying all the things I'd said to patients over the years about bad pathology results. None of those carefully chosen words seemed remotely adequate now that I was on the receiving end of them.

BREAKING THE RULES

Day six post-surgery and I was done being a good patient. *The Handmaid's Tale* had gotten too dark to watch without Tracy, my kids were at school, and everyone was working. The house felt like it was shrinking around me.

When I suggested to a friend that we go see the manatees and he readily agreed to drive, I felt like I was getting out of jail. "Are you sure?" he questioned before I got into his car, reasonably concerned about taking a fresh post-op patient on an excursion.

"Yeah, why not?" I said . . . as if I hadn't spent years telling patients *exactly* why not. "My legs still work; I just can't swing my arms when I walk. Fresh air will do me good. Besides, you can't even tell I have drains in." I twirled around in an oversize shirt.

Sabrina had clearly reminded me about the importance of restricting movement in my arms and torso. "When you move your chest wall, you're creating a shearing effect," she explained as she slid the palms of her hands up and down against each other. "In order for the reconstruction to be successful, the surface of the implant needs to stick to your tissue. Any excessive movement will create this shearing effect and can lead to implant failure. Monitoring your drain output will give me an idea of how well you're listening to me. The less movement, the less shearing, the less fluid." The explanation made total sense, and I had told my patients the same thing countless times. But it was different for me because I knew that if I just walked like a T-rex, keeping my arms tight by my side, I could minimize chest wall movement. I was so smart!

Bad Sue!

By day eight, having suffered no physical setbacks from my manatee adventure and thoroughly sick of my recliner, I decided to go hiking. Yes, hiking. Eight days postmastectomy. It was a cool, brisk day and walking was exactly what I thought I needed.

As I was about to start the trail, Devina called. I wasn't going to answer because I didn't want to tell her where I was (also I'm a horrible liar). But if I didn't answer, she would have driven over to my house to make sure I was still alive.

"Hey there," I said nonchalantly.

"How are you feeling?"

"Fine. I'm fine." I assured her.

"I'll be over in an hour, okay? Do you need me to bring anything?"

"Uh, I'm not home," I replied quietly.

"What are you doing?" she demanded to know. I told her my plans like a child caught red-handed.

"You can't be doing this! Sabrina is going to kill you, and then she's going to kill me for letting you do this." She was getting more and more pissed off as she spoke. "Are you aware that most people take six weeks off after the surgery and rest? You are already pushing it by planning to go back to work next week!"

But I was already on my way, T-rex walk activated.

The consequences of my rebellion soon showed up in the drain output. The fluid that should have been decreasing stayed steady, and the drains that should have come out at two weeks stayed in longer. When I went for my two-week follow-up, Sabrina asked, "What are you doing?"

"Nothing," I lied. "Watching TV, maybe going for a little walk."

Sabrina was clearly frustrated. She stepped out of the room and texted Lisa and Devina: "I don't know how many more ways I can say this to get it through her thick skull. She really needs to not move. Anything you guys can say will help."

Devina, meanwhile, was thinking, *Oh, I should probably not tell Sabrina that Sue went on a five-mile hike yesterday.*

When Sabrina re-entered the room, she sat down on her stool and scooted toward me. "Sue," she started. She spoke differently. There was no friendly undertone; it was more of a *We are going to have a come-to-Jesus moment right now* inflection. "Most patients have drains pulled at two weeks. You are not ready, but here's the thing. I will only allow these to stay in one more week because after that your risk of infection really starts to climb. And if you get an infection, you run the risk of implant failure. Listen really carefully to me right now. If your implant fails, you will need another surgery, another recovery, and another round of restrictions. I know the doctor in you understands this, but the Sue in you is clearly having a problem coming to terms with being a patient. You are a patient right now, and you need to be for the next few days. Please," she pleaded.

I walked out of my two-week follow-up with Sabrina with my head down and completely ashamed and embarrassed. I thought I could be the exception with all my advanced knowledge, but all my knowledge ended up giving me a false sense of invincibility and making me one of *those* patients who doctors dread dealing with. While I knew fully from all my years of practice that breast cancer was nondiscriminatory, I had to become a more obedient patient to learn that no one is exempt from the rules of recovery. After I left the appointment, I told myself I needed to behave and start listening to my doctors and adhering to their advice.

The whole situation put my medical team in an impossible position. These were my colleagues, my friends, trying to treat a doctor who thought she knew better. And I was a doctor becoming the kind of patient that I found most challenging. But sometimes the best lessons come from being on the other side of medical advice, from learning firsthand why those restrictions exist, and from finally understanding that medical knowledge doesn't make you immune to the fundamental rules of healing.

I finally accepted what I had always told my patients: Recovery isn't a race. You can't rush healing. Your body will heal at its own pace, but only if you let it.

WHEN REALITY SHIFTS

Looking back on those early days of recovery—from the funeral home atmosphere of my flower-filled house to the moment we learned the full pathology results—certain truths emerged that would shape the rest of my journey.

First, there was the overwhelming show of support. Every wilting flower and empty casserole dish and every friend sleeping by my bedside, visiting, cleaning, calling, and texting represented someone sincerely offering help. The challenge wasn't finding support, it was learning to receive it gracefully.

Then there was my rebellion against recovery restrictions. How many times had I told patients to take it easy so their bodies had all the necessary resources to heal? Yet there I was six days post-surgery hanging out with manatees. Eight days post-surgery I went hiking. The drains that wouldn't stop draining told their own story about the cost of not listening.

Humor became my lifeline. The Boobie Fairy's visit, my kids feeding me Cheetos and Takis as I dozed in and out of consciousness, friends taking selfies with me snoring away in my recliner obliviously in the background—these moments of levity punctuated the darkness. Sometimes laughter is the only sensible response to the insensible reality of cancer.

But perhaps the most profound theme was the complete dissolution of my boundaries. The lines between professional and personal blurred beyond recognition. Lisa retired and then returned a few days later to offer me help. Sabrina texted my friends for help with my drain output. Julie cleaned my house while I ate ice cream and waited for pathology results.

The treatment plan's escalation from what we thought would be a straightforward surgery to include chemotherapy and radiation forced me to confront my own mortality in ways I hadn't expected. As a doctor, I knew all the statistics, all the treatment protocols, all the potential outcomes. As a patient, I had to learn to live with daunting uncertainty.

Moving forward meant accepting a new reality: that my knowledge would not protect me from fear and that being a doctor definitely did not make me a better patient. It meant acknowledging that the path ahead would be longer and harder than I'd hoped. The lessons of those early recovery days would always stay with me: healing isn't linear, support comes in many amazing forms, and the best medicine is letting others care for me, even when (especially when) it makes me uncomfortable.

As I faced the next phase of treatment, I carried these lessons with me and found a new kind of strength—not in being perfect, but in being a vulnerable human; not in knowing all the answers, but in being willing to face the questions; not in maintaining control, but in learning to let go. The path ahead would require everything I had learned as a doctor and everything I was learning as a patient. My house might have looked like someone died, but it wasn't about death. It was about my messy, imperfect, supported, beloved life. And that was what I was willing to fight for.

Chapter Five

SECOND OPINIONS
AND FIRST DAYS

" I feel like I'm cheating on him," I confessed to my sister, who called and advised me to see another oncologist to confirm my treatment plan.

"I know Wassim is your colleague, but you need to get a second opinion. Remember I'm a breast radiologist, so I know what I'm talking about. He won't be offended, people do it all the time. When my friend was diagnosed, she went to Dana Farber and she also thinks you should go there too." By the tone in her voice, I knew this was not a request. Ever since I got diagnosed, Min had been hounding me to go outside of my system and get another opinion.

Second opinions are very common in cancer care, and when a patient asks me if it's okay, I encourage it. The last thing I want my patients to worry about is whether I am doing things correctly. But this was different because it was Wassim, my friend and my colleague of five years, whom I trusted implicitly. He was well respected and connected. While I didn't like his recommendation for me, I understood the basis for it. I also knew that all others agreed with his plan, since Devina and Tracy polled every medical oncologist they knew. Everyone had variations on how to look at the pathology, but in the end the recommendation was always the same.

My sister refused to back down, so finally I agreed. It would be a twenty-four-hour trip, and Wassim would never know the better.

"Fine! I'll do it." I yelled back and hung up. Within the hour, she had the Dana Farber scheduling department calling to set up an appointment. I was instructed to be there on February 14th, Valentine's Day, at 3:30 PM. Lisa offered to come with me, and I welcomed the company. I knew not many patients show up to their appointments with their surgeon in tow, so I considered myself extremely fortunate. Having her there would allow us to have a multidisciplinary discussion, with me giving radiation input even though I was the patient.

I called my sister back to let her know the appointment was confirmed.

"I'm glad to hear this," she said victoriously. "I'll definitely feel more comfortable after you're seen at Dana Farber, and I'm sure you'll feel more comfortable too."

The truth? I wasn't comfortable with any of it. I wasn't comfortable with my diagnosis, with my pathology results, with the mounting evidence that my cancer was more complex than we'd initially thought. And I *definitely* wasn't comfortable going behind Wassim's back to get another opinion.

But I did it anyway to keep peace with my sister.

THE SECRET JOURNEY

"I'll meet you at the airport," I told Lisa confidently.

"Sue, you can't drive."

"What?"

"You had surgery ten days ago. You can't drive. Did you even read Sabrina's post-op instructions?" Lisa questioned.

I hadn't but it really did slip my mind that I was still on driving restrictions until Lisa reminded me. That's how scattered I was. Lisa ended up driving me to the airport, probably wondering how someone who'd spent her career treating breast cancer patients could be such a difficult patient herself.

The journey to Boston felt surreal. The weather was freezing—a shock to my Florida system—but that wasn't what made me shiver as we approached the imposing building. Walking into one of the country's premier cancer centers as a patient felt different from walking into *my* hospital as a patient. At Dana Farber, no one knew me as a doctor, so I was treated like everyone else. At my hospital, everyone knew who I was, so the staff was always a little bit more personal in our interactions. The efficiency of their system, which I'd normally appreciate from a professional standpoint, now processed me like any other scared patient seeking answers. Upon checking in, the receptionist handed me a tracker to record how quickly I moved through the appointment. During the intake, the medical assistants and nurses used layman's terms when asking me questions. I answered yes or no, giving them no clue that I had any medical expertise.

We were then led to a patient room and the medical oncologist entered before we could even sit down. He had a warmth and kindness to him that put me immediately at ease. Sometimes doctors at the top of their field can be condescending and unapproachable, but he was quite the opposite. Despite his impressive credentials, he questioned me like a medical student, asking me to elaborate on every little detail and writing down my answers on his notepad. His thoroughness in taking my history was surpassed by his detailed explanation of his recommendation. I felt like I was sitting in a residency journal club as we reviewed the publications that provided the rationale for his decision-making. As a resident, I could barely stay awake when inundated with so much data. But as a patient, I eagerly absorbed everything he told me.

I appreciated being treated like any other patient with a complicated case, seeking answers. It was the first time I was truly able to detach the doctor side of me from the patient side of me, which is exactly how it needed to be in order for me to start coming to terms with my new identity as a cancer patient.

"You are clinically high risk, but the genetics of your tumor are low risk if you trust MammaPrint, but intermediate risk if you trust Oncotype," he summarized as we were coming toward the end of the consultation. "The benefit of chemotherapy for you is likely from it shutting down your ovaries because your tumor is so responsive to estrogen, so chemotherapy is not wrong in your situation. But you would likely get the same benefit from Lupron, which I saw you already received. In terms of radiation, I know you know the data better than me, but I would definitely give you radiation. There are too many red flags in your pathology report, and I am concerned about your risk of local recurrence if you don't do it. But you are the expert when it comes to this, so I defer this decision to you. Because you are hormone receptor-positive, you need to be on endocrine therapy. Your positive lymph node also makes you a candidate for CDK4/6 inhibitors, and by the time you're done with definitive treatment, there will be new data published to support this."

"When you say I'd 'likely get the same benefit with Lupron,' how likely is that likely?" When I realized it was a confusing question with all those likelys, I rephrased it. "So you are saying I don't need to do chemo?"

"What scares you more?" he asked, leaning forward slightly, "The side effects of chemotherapy or the prospect of metastatic disease?"

It was the kind of question I'd asked patients hundreds of times. But hearing him ask me that question felt different. In my head, I understood what he was saying. But in my heart? In my heart, I was just scared of dying from this cancer. I've met too many patients who weren't supposed to fail but did. Caring for these women at the end of their lives as they died slow, painful deaths always took an emotional toll on me, even though I managed to maintain professional on the outside. While many of the patients seemed to have accepted their fate at the end of their lives, their family members—the ones who would have to learn to live without them—were often the ones who pushed their worn-down bodies to keep fighting. I thought of my boys and wanted to do everything possible to protect them from that.

"I want to trust the results of the Mammaprint and would feel so much better if I also got a low risk Oncotype. I realize all the tumors in my breast likely have the same biology but I wish we could run genomics on all the tumors to confirm none of them are high risk . . ." He nodded his head in agreement.

"I can live with side effects," I replied. "I don't want to die of metastatic disease."

"Okay, well there's our answer." He turned back to the notepad to jot a quick note about our discussion.

"What's my prognosis?" It was a question that I knew the answer to but still wanted to ask. I wanted someone else to confirm what I knew. Wassim didn't talk about numbers at all with me. He just kept telling me I would be fine, and I never had the courage to ask. Now I did.

"Are you sure you want to talk numbers?" he asked.

"Yes. I know we went over the data and the relative benefit, but I'm asking you to tell me an absolute number."

Then came the number: "Ten-year survival, eighty-five percent."

Unexpectedly, I broke down in his office. Hearing my own survival statistics hit differently. While I knew eighty-five percent was very high, I consider breast cancer patients to be the overachievers of the cancer population with outcomes of ninety-five to ninety-nine percent for those with early-stage disease. Hearing that I couldn't hit at least ninety percent with chemotherapy, endocrine therapy and CDK4/6 inhibitors was a crushing blow. A fifteen percent chance of dying in ten years was a shock to my system. Suddenly, I wasn't calculating odds—I was living them.

BACK TO REALITY

Two weeks post-surgery, I returned to work. I still had drains in, which I strategically hid under a carefully chosen loose-fitting white button-down collared shirt from Target. I figured if I looked good, I could convince myself that I felt good too. In addition, I needed to get out of my recliner and back into reality because I felt like my brain was slowly dissolving.

I can manage this, I thought as I parked my car outside my office. Walking into the building felt surreal. Everything looked exactly the same—the same desk, same chairs, same diplomas on the wall. But *I* wasn't the same. For one, my physical limitations were obvious. I couldn't get my arms above my head to demonstrate proper positioning for radiation for the patients. I couldn't be as hands-on when I had patients on the planning table and had to rely more on my radiation therapists for help. I couldn't ignore the fact that I had drains because they rubbed against the exit sites of my chest wall anytime I moved. But the psychological challenges were harder to navigate: How do you counsel patients about their cancer journey when you're in the middle of your own?

My first consultation was a healthy seventy-five-year-old female who looked like she was in her late fifties. She didn't have any medical issues and underwent a mammogram for routine screening. The imaging showed Stage I breast cancer. Her tumor was ER positive and HER2 negative. She decided to undergo a lumpectomy and scheduled an appointment with me to hear about her radiation options. I started my discussion just as I had done countless times before, explaining what the stage meant, what the pathology report said, and the significance of her receptor status.

"For early-stage breast cancer, a lumpectomy followed by radiation is essentially the same as a mastectomy in terms of outcome. So whether or not you choose to remove the entire breast or preserve your breast and add radiation, you are going to do the same," I explained.

She nodded her head in understanding. I continued, "Since that data has been published, we've learned that there are some patients who will have good control with a lumpectomy alone."

I apparently piqued her interest because she perked up and started listening more intently. "For women over the age of seventy with favorable tumor profiles like your own, a lumpectomy alone will give you a ninety percent chance of local control, and if you add radiation, that number will increase to ninety-eight percent. Radiation will not affect your survival."

"So I don't need radiation?" she questioned.

"The benefit of radiation may not be clinically significant to you. Meaning that radiation will take you from an A minus to an A plus, but will that better grade impact you in the long run? Probably not. As my eleven-year-old loves to tell me, 'Mom, Cs get degrees!'" I chuckled as I thought of Nathan. "More importantly, you will continue getting mammograms every year at a minimum. If something does come back, it will likely be caught early, and we can treat you with another lumpectomy and radiation at that time and call it a day."

My last statement, something I've said repeatedly to other patients in the same situation over the years, stopped me in my tracks. I thought of my situation. I went for my mammograms every year, but my cancer wasn't caught early. I knew that my case was considered a "one-off," but how could I continue to recommend no radiation and have confidence in my recommendation based on my personal experience? After what I'd been through, I was tempted to treat everyone because it really sucked to be the "one-off."

I thought of the few patients who ended up recurring several years later after they elected to hold off on radiation. The psychological implications of their cancer returning were devastating for some, as they beat themselves up for not pursuing all the treatment when they were initially diagnosed. Before I was the one with cancer, I did my best to comfort them and reassure them that they made the right decision, fully knowing that there is no such thing as a guarantee. Now that I had cancer, I wanted to treat everyone because the fear of recurrence was so pervasive for me that I wanted to spare anyone I could from that experience.

At the end of our appointment, the patient asked me, "Doc, what would you do if you were me?" Patients always asked me this question, but this was my first time hearing it since being diagnosed. *I am you*, I thought in my head. I went back and forth about whether I should regurgitate my precancer answer, "It's a very personal choice, and the decision to pursue radiation is based on the anxiety level of the patient." Now that I was in the thick of cancer treatment, I realized how wimpy that answer was. These patients sought guidance, and I would leave the ball in their court and let them make the decision. My diagnosis forced me to re-evaluate my approach to patients. Should I be honest about how my personal experience could be clouding my judgement? Would I be able to ever approach a breast cancer patient objectively again? Old habits die hard, so I spat out my precancer answer. Much to my relief, the patient wanted to err on the side of caution and opted for radiation.

I managed to make it through the first two days of work without any major issues. On my drive home, I answered some calls from referring doctors who asked if I was back, and I responded enthusiastically, "I'm back and open for business!"

As soon as I got home, I went to the bathroom to empty my drains. I unpinned the bulb from my bra and looked at the fluid level. Given that I spent most of my day talking to patients and not moving very much, I was surprised that the bulb was almost full. The last time the bulb was that full was right after my hike. This was a major setback for me. I had five more days before Sabrina was going to pull the drains, regardless of what the output read. While I was mentally ready to get back to work, physically it was another story. I dialed Julie.

"Hey, Sue," she answered cheerfully. "How are you feeling?"

"I need the rest of the week off," I said, crying softly.

"It's okay. It's going to be okay. What's going on?"

"My output," I sniffled. "There's too much drain output today. I think it's from working the past two days. There's too much."

"Not a problem," she responded quickly. "You have double coverage for the next few weeks for this reason." She paused for a minute. "Sue, maybe you need a few more weeks off?"

"No, it's too depressing in the house, and chemo will start in two weeks. I need to get back to working. It is the only thing that makes me feel normal right now."

I climbed back into my recliner and stayed put for the next five days. My output dropped to less than five milliliters when I returned to Sabrina's office. "Perfect," she said with a satisfied and relieved look as she pulled the long drains out of my chest wall.

THE SUPPORT SQUAD MOBILIZES

With surgery several weeks behind me and physical restrictions lifted, I started to feel more human and regain my independence. Slowly but surely, I was on the road to recovery from the mastectomies. But now I had to focus on the treatment that lay ahead. It was easier for me to come to terms with needing chemotherapy than it was radiation. While chemotherapy scared me, radiation terrified me because I knew too much. I'd seen every possible complication, managed every potential side effect, and handled every worst-case scenario. It was hard not to see my face on those who had their reconstructions severely compromised by radiation.

In terms of where to get treatment, I knew Wassim would supervise my chemotherapy. But what about radiation? I'd always wondered, in a vague way, where I would go for radiation if I ever needed it. Now I had to actually make that decision. Would the staff that I'd spent the past ten years training find it awkward as I lay topless on their table? Would my partner be comfortable treating me? I didn't know the answer to these questions, but I couldn't imagine going anywhere else. If I had to do radiation, I wanted it done in my department with the people I trusted.

Chemotherapy would be first. Once Wassim got insurance authorization, he sent me a schedule.

"March 6th," he told me. "Be at the infusion center at 7:30 AM. My office will call in your pre-medications. Make sure you get the prescriptions and take them as directed. I mean it, Sue. For you to tolerate chemo with minimal side effects, you have to take everything EXACTLY as I prescribe it." He spoke slowly and enunciated every word clearly, as if to ensure that he wouldn't be to blame if I decided to deviate from the plan.

I laughed out loud because he was talking the way I talked to my children when I knew they weren't going to listen.

"This isn't funny," he said sternly, not finding humor in any of this. "You didn't listen very well to Sabrina, and you're lucky that you didn't develop complications. I know how sick patients can get from chemo. I don't want that to be you, and I know you don't want that to be you."

"I get it, Wassim. Anything else?"

"I saw you got a second opinion," he finally said. *Crap*, I thought to myself. I knew I should have told him, but I chickened out because I didn't want to hurt his feelings. "I wanted your pathology slides sent to Mayo for a second opinion and was surprised when I found out they were sent to Dana Farber."

"I was going to tell you about that," I started. "My sister is a doctor, and she wouldn't stop harassing me until I got another opinion. I didn't know how you would take it."

"You know, when I asked Devina, she took the blame for your second opinion and didn't mention anything about your sister." He paused for a few seconds. "Listen, I don't care who you see. I just wish you would have told me."

The irony wasn't lost on me—here we were, all these highly trained medical professionals, playing out an almost adolescent-like drama of secret-keeping and hurt feelings. But cancer has a way of stripping away professional pretense, leaving just our human vulnerabilities exposed.

Now that I had a schedule, my support system kicked into high gear. Julie arranged for my clinic schedule to be extremely light the first few days after chemotherapy. Tracy planned her return trip so that she could sit by my side for the first infusion. Devina explained to my kids why I needed more treatment and begged them to get along or at least fake it for my sake. Marie reactivated the meal train to come at the start of every cycle. James got his driver's license and offered to drive his brothers when I didn't feel up to it.

While the path forward wasn't what I'd hoped for, at least there was a path. Chemotherapy. Radiation. CDK4/6 inhibitors in addition to the endocrine therapy that was initially planned. It was a lot. It was overwhelming. But it was also a plan, and having a plan meant having something to focus on besides fear.

That night, I sat in my recliner looking at all the flowers—now in the final stage of life—and thought about how many times I'd delivered news like this to patients. How many times I'd outlined aggressive treatment plans and watched their faces fall. How many times I'd assured them they could handle it. Now I was the one who needed to believe that. The journey forward wasn't the one I'd wanted, but it was the one I had. And the only way out was through.

PREPARING FOR BATTLE

The two features that people immediately notice about me when they meet me are my height and my hair. Because I'm Asian, everyone expects me to be short, so it's always a bit of a shock when I enter a room at five foot, eight inches. The concept of a tall Asian is apparently an oxymoron. I inevitably get asked if I get my height from my parents, which I don't with both standing at only five feet tall.

My parents do, however, have really great heads of hair, and thanks to them, I also have truly beautiful hair. It was brownish-black with a slight wave to it and flowed down to my mid-back. The texture was smooth and soft, having never dyed it before. My hairstylist called it her "dream hair." I even had a patient once tell me, "What do you know about bad hair? You have porn star hair!" as I tried to console her because her hair did not grow back the same after chemo.

When I learned I would be getting chemo, the one side effect that scared me the most was the hair loss because I didn't know how to be me without my hair. Luckily, the infusion center where I would be receiving treatment had just gotten a cold capping system, and I would be the first one to use it.

"The key to effective hair preservation is getting the cap to fit tightly," the nurse explained as she pulled out a small blue cap for me to try on. Channels ran throughout the cap in a pattern that resembled the outside contour of the human brain. *Well, this is an interesting design,* I thought to myself as I took the cap and tried to imagine sitting through chemo with it on. As a doctor, I knew the science behind cold capping—the cold constricts blood vessels in the scalp, preventing chemotherapy from reaching the hair follicles. As a patient, I saw a means to self-preservation.

Like anything in medicine, there was no guarantee it would work, but it was the best option. This was where having thick hair was going to work in my favor—because I had so much, I could lose most of it and still look like I had a full head of hair. My thick hair, however, also made the small cap feel like a tight vice around my head. There was no way I would be able to endure an hour with it on. I swapped it out for the medium cap, which fit much better.

"That was easy," she said as she tested the fit by trying to slip a finger between the cap and my head. "Medium is the right size. I'll have Doc sign off on the order. Once you call the company with your credit card, they will FedEx the supplies to your house. Bring the kit with you to the first day of chemo. Oh, and go online to the company's website. They have some pretty helpful videos on how to use the cap."

With the cap figured out, I turned my attention to my eyebrows . . . yes, my eyebrows. It may seem like a weird thing to think about when heading into chemo, but they are hair, and just like the hair on your head, eyebrows can thin or fall out. If I was going to put the effort into cold capping to preserve what was on my head, then I also needed to do something to preserve my eyebrows. Having a good head of hair without any eyebrows would more or less defeat the purpose.

I was fortunate to have Heather in my village. I first met her when our kids were assigned to the same flag football team. She was naturally artistic and the go-to person for anything creative, like the end of the season coaching gifts. Eventually, she used her abilities to start a microblading business that quickly became extremely popular simply through word of mouth. When she found out about my diagnosis, she texted to let me know she was praying for me and to let her know if I needed anything. Knowing that she always booked out way in advance, I jokingly texted back, "How about microblading . . . lol." "Absolutely, just let me know when you are available!" she responded immediately. Within a few days, she slipped me into her schedule and got my eyebrows ready for chemo by tattooing on ones that looked so real that no one would be the wiser when the real ones fell out.

Next on my list was preventing neuropathy. According to Wassim, the chances that I would get neuropathy from chemo were low, but I wasn't going to risk it. Neuropathy is a condition where damage to the nerves results in pain, numbness, tingling, and/or weakness. One of my colleagues, who developed the condition when she received chemo for breast cancer, had to go on permanent disability because she couldn't feel as well when she was operating. I've also had multiple patients suffer bad falls that resulted in hospital stays in the orthopedic unit because the neuropathy in their feet made them so unsteady. *An ounce of prevention is worth a pound of* cure, I thought to myself as I went onto Amazon to order ice mitts and socks to wear during the Taxotere infusion. They worked in the same way as the cold cap, causing the blood vessels in my hands and feet to constrict, thereby minimizing the amount of chemotherapy to those areas.

In terms of work life accommodations, I anticipated minimal disruption. I had four cycles of chemotherapy prescribed with three weeks between every cycle. Treatment would be given on day one, which happened to coincide with my admin day. The following day I foresaw feeling great because I would still be pumped up on steroids, which Wassim instructed me to take the day before, the day of, and the day after chemo to prevent nausea. Friday, Saturday, and Sunday would be my down days and then, if everything went as planned, I would be good as new by Monday. Repeat three times and then move on to radiation.

Julie encouraged me to take more time off, but I said no. I wanted my normal back. I wanted my busy clinic of patients. I wanted to be running around the hospital complaining about how I hated running around the hospital. I wanted to rush off to James's high school so that I could watch some of his baseball game. I wanted to make it to Chick-fil-A just before they closed so that I wouldn't have to worry about cooking dinner. I wanted to go home, pass out for the evening, then wake up and repeat the same routine the next day. I wanted all of it.

My precancer pride was still going strong. Now that I was well on the road to recovering from surgery, I convinced myself that I would be able to fly through chemotherapy with my carefully crafted schedule.

I spent the final few days leading up to chemo immersed in my typical routine: work, boys, sleep, wake-up, and repeat. As I got further out from surgery and more into my precancer routine, I felt my old self coming back. And then someone would ask me (always with the best of intentions) how I was feeling and if I needed anything, and I would instantly be brought back into my current reality of fake boobs and breast cancer.

When I finished seeing patients the day before my first cycle, I went to my office and tidied up, a ritual I typically did when I was going to be out of the office for a prolonged period of time. I opened my office fridge and out wafted a horrible smell that indicated something was clearly decaying in there. Holding my nose, I threw everything out and left the door open. I went through a stack of mail and trashed junk journals that were piling up on the corner of my desk. I wiped down my phone, keyboard, mouse, and desktop.

"Are you planning to be gone for a while?" Marie asked as she witnessed me stuffing papers into an already full trash can. "You know you're scheduled to come in on Monday, right?"

"I know," I responded without looking up. "But I kind of feel like, as much as I've been trying to resist this thought, the old me isn't coming back. Everything is different . . . I'm different," I said leaning back in my desk chair, looking around my office. "Patients come through our doors and get treatment every day, and I've never thought much about how the treatment might change them."

"But we all do this," Marie offered in an understanding tone. "If we get personal with all our patients, we wouldn't be able to survive this job. You know that as well as I do."

"I know. I just wonder if I'm doing my patients a disservice by not acknowledging this."

"You would be doing your patient a disservice by getting too involved. You need to stay one step removed to maintain your objectivity."

"How do I remain objective when I can see myself in the patients now?" I questioned.

Marie didn't have an answer and I didn't expect her to. She gave me a hug, wished me luck with chemo, and shut my office door behind her.

After weeks of being strong and trying to maintain some semblance of control, I broke down in tears as I sat alone in my nicely tidied office. I didn't want to be known as a breast cancer patient. I didn't want to have chemo. I didn't want to have radiation. I didn't want to be sick. I didn't want to be tired. But above all, I didn't want to die of cancer—and that trumped everything else I didn't want.

I got in my car and started the ignition. I looked at my reflection in the rearview mirror—the doctor who'd thought she knew everything about breast cancer until she was diagnosed with cancer.

"One day at a time," I whispered to my reflection. This was what I always told my patients. Maybe it was time to take my own advice.

The final preparations for chemotherapy felt both methodical and surreal. Tracy flew in again to support me through the first cycle. After I picked her up from the airport, we went to the pharmacy to grab all the medications Wassim prescribed and then set alarms on my phone to remind me to take them. The treatment calendar stretched out before me like a road map to a destination I never wanted to visit. Training for a marathon would have been easier—at least then you know where the finish line is. With cancer treatment, each finish line just leads to another starting point. After surgery, there would be chemo. After chemo, there would be radiation, After radiation, there would be CDK4/6 inhibitors and endocrine therapy. Each phase brings its own challenges, its own fears, its own opportunities to either break down or break through.

"Are you ready?" Tracy asked, helping me organize my chemo bag with the cold cap, ice mitts and socks, blankets, snacks, and my work laptop.

Ready? How could anyone ever be ready? But I nodded anyway. Because that's what you do. You nod and say you're ready, even when you're not.

"You got this," Tracy said with the kind of certainty I used to have when I said those words to my patients.

I spent the last night of phase one wandering through the house. All signs of surgery had been cleared from the bathroom countertops and replaced with prescription bottles that were lined up by height. The kids and dogs were fast asleep. I, on the other hand, was wide awake thanks to the steroids I took earlier to prevent nausea. Sleeping was not in the cards so rather than fight it, I went with the flow. For the next six hours, I folded all the laundry, cleaned the fish tank and then reorganized the laundry room, master closet, and pantry. Just as I was throwing out a can of beans that expired five years ago, Zeus came into the kitchen for breakfast.

"Guess it's time for me to get ready?" I asked Zeus as he stood there, eagerly wagging his tail, excited to eat.

After I fed the dogs, I headed to my bathroom to get ready. Phase two was about to begin. Ready or not, here I go.

Chapter Six
CHEMOTHERAPY CHRONICLES

*P*lease don't let me run into any patients in the lobby.

That was my first thought walking into the infusion center, scanning the faces to see if anyone was my patient. I thought about the times I sat in the radiology holding room with patients whose mammograms I'd ordered. When they recognized me, they would exclaim, "Dr. Hwang!" which would always trigger other patients in the holding area to look at me. Their anxiety was always greater than mine because they were the ones who had cancer (at the time), and I would distract them with small talk and gentle reassurance. I thought about this as I entered the infusion center's waiting room. On this day, I just wanted to be a normal patient seeking healthcare. I was nervous enough already and didn't have the bandwidth for small talk or the strength to encourage others.

Now, as a patient, each step felt like a potential collision between worlds. I knew exactly where I was going, of course. Down the hall, past the staff lounge, last room in the back. But today, I had to check in at the front desk, sit in the waiting room, and wait for the nurse to call my name. I had to be processed like any other patient starting chemotherapy. HGTV played on the

TV as I waited to be called, prompting flashbacks to the day I was diagnosed. As I sat there watching another home be demolished, more patients checked in and soon every seat was occupied. I didn't want to shift my gaze away from the TV for fear of making eye contact with anyone in the waiting room, on the chance that they were my patient.

"Sue?" a nurse finally called out. I shot up and hurried toward her. Tracy followed with bags and pastries in tow. "I'm actually going to take you the back way, so we don't have to walk through the entire infusion center. We will do our best to protect your privacy."

I was placed in a room separate from the other patients—one that was considerably larger to accommodate the cold capping system. Roughly the size of a small mini-fridge, the machine was positioned to the right of the infusion chair. An IV pole that hung a full bag of saline was located to the left of the chair, and the chemo chair itself was a simple recliner, functional but unremarkable.

Once we got settled, Tracy held out a box of baked goods that we picked up that morning to ensure they would be fresh because no one likes a stale pastry. "Anyone want Panera? We have muffins, cookies, and croissants," she announced, like bribing the staff with pastries was a completely normal part of the chemotherapy protocol. Then again, maybe it was. I'd never been on this side of it before, but I knew how happy my staff became when patients came with treats—it always made them smile and laugh a little bit more and reminded them that they were appreciated.

The nurse drew my blood and inserted an IV into my left arm. She then injected medications to prevent nausea and an infusion reaction. Fifteen minutes later, she returned and informed me, "Your counts are good, so we'll order your chemo from the pharmacy now. Get prepped for the cold cap," and she pulled the curtain shut behind her.

Tracy pulled out a spray bottle of water and started wetting down my hair. We quickly moved to the bathroom because water was getting all over the floor of the infusion room. She continued to spray and then finally exclaimed, "Just stick your head under the faucet. You have way too much hair for the spray bottle to handle and my hand is starting to cramp."

I couldn't help but burst out laughing. Here I was about to start my first cycle of chemotherapy, and I'm sticking my head under the faucet like I did when I was ten years old. Except back then I did it to convince my parents that I'd showered when I really hadn't.

"Are you sure about this?" I asked her as she turned on the water.

"Yes. I watched the video last night, and we have to make sure your hair is wet so the cap can effectively conduct the cold to your scalp. Come on, bend over." She ran her fingers through my hair and ensured everything was drenched. When I came out of the bathroom, I looked as if I was at a hair salon, with one towel draped over my shoulders and another draped over my head.

I returned to the recliner and Tracy got out a bottle of leave-in conditioner, squirting a dime size amount into the palm on my hand. "Okay, you need a thin layer. It's just to help the cold cap glide on."

"Thank God you are here. I wouldn't know how to do this without you."

"I know. And I know you definitely didn't watch those videos that were recommended, which is why I stayed up last night watching them." She knew me too well. I tended to figure things out on the fly, whereas she would carefully read instructions several times over and follow them exactly. She grabbed the inner lining of the cold cap and slid it over my hair. She then stretched the outer liner of the cap, which served to insulate the inside cap, and positioned it on my head. Once she confirmed everything was good and snug, she snapped the buckle under my chin closed. "Okay," she informed the nurse. "We are ready to get hooked up."

The nurse looked at us with hesitation. "Uh, I'm going to be honest, you are the first patient we've used this on. We had an in-service from the device rep yesterday, but we are going to have to figure this out together. Let me go get the manual."

As a patient, there was nothing reassuring about this moment. I didn't want to make a big deal about the nurse's self-declared inexperience because this was just about hair preservation, but I paid a lot of money for cold capping and I *really* did not want to lose my hair. As providers, we all have firsts with our patients, but we don't typically make it known because no patient wants to be someone's first.

I remember the first consult I did as an attending physician, the first time I treated a patient by myself, and the first time I contaminated my patient's lead contact lens, which I accidentally dropped on the floor as I was trying to place it over his eye to protect the eye from radiation. I was a resident at the time, and as the lens hit the floor, the entire room fell silent and the senior radiation therapist gave me a look that said, "*Oooooooh, you are in trouble now. The attending will be here any minute to check the set-up, and you just contaminated the protective shield.*"

Not wanting to panic the patient, I calmly told the therapist, "I want to use a larger lens. Can you please get it for me?" I held this lens tightly between my thumb and forefinger, and as I spread the patient's upper and lower lid apart, I slid it over the eye, praying that it would fit. And it did. It was actually a better fit so we ended up using it for the remainder of the patient's treatment. Afterwards, the therapist pulled me aside to tell me how impressed he was with my ability to problem solve in the moment without letting the patient know that there was an issue. By staying calm, I was able to ensure that the patient maintained a high level of confidence in the treatment team.

The nurse returned with the start-up guide in hand. As I sat in the chair, Tracy and the nurse ran through the directions. They took the two tubes that came from the back of the cap and connected them to the tubing from the cold capping system, which was a compact refrigeration unit that circulated coolant through the cap.

"Key fob?" Tracy asked. I pointed to one of the bags on the floor. She dug around and after a minute pulled out a small oval-shaped fob. She pressed it against the machine and hit the start button. Instantly, I heard fluid gushing through the cap, and within a few minutes, the periphery of my scalp felt very, very cold.

"This is the pre-infusion cooling phase. During this phase, the temperature of your scalp is slowly being brought down," the nurse read to me. "After this is complete, there will be a treatment cycle and then a post-infusion phase. Okay," she sighed as she put down the manual. "That wasn't that hard at all. I'm going to see where the pharmacy is with filling your chemo order."

The nurse returned twenty minutes later with a bag of chemotherapy in hand. "First, a time-out, and then we start the infusion." Once my name, date of birth, name of chemo, and dose were confirmed, she hung the bag on the IV pole and connected it to my line. She rolled open the IV lock, and I watched as the chemo slowly dripped into the tubing and then eventually into my left arm. Phase two had officially begun.

Tracy pulled out her laptop and rummaged through my bag for mine. She handed me my computer, which I promptly opened. Together, we sat there working side by side, just as we did in the old days when we staffed the same clinic. The depth of our friendship was shown by our ability to sit in a small room together, each doing our own thing, with no concerns about awkward silence.

"One bag done, one more to go," the nurse announced after an hour. She took down the empty bag and left to get the second bag of chemo.

Tracy said as she put her computer away, "Let's get the mitts and socks on."

Lisa had arrived by this time, and she and Tracy treated me like a toddler as they put frozen mitts on my hands and socks on my feet. The mitts resembled oven mitts, or for baseball fans out there, sliding mitts. I sat in the recliner with my hands and feet in the air and shot both of them a huge grin. "I must look amazing right now, right?" I asked giggling.

Tracy burst out laughing and grabbed her phone. "Just one picture, for posterity's sake."

The nurse performed her second time-out and then hung the next bag of chemo. "Halfway through," she said with encouragement. She opened the line, and the second chemo started running into my IV. Almost instantly, I felt a burning coursing through the vein in my arm. *Wow, that burns!* I didn't want to say anything because I didn't want to be *that* patient—the one that becomes known for complaining. *Count for a few seconds and the burning will go away . . . one . . . two . . . three . . . four . . .* The pain got worse, though. I started running through the differential in my head, wondering if the chemotherapy was leaking into the surrounding tissue. It's called extravasation, and it happens occasionally. As the chemo leaks, it causes a chemical burn in the surrounding tissue. I looked at my arm but didn't see any indication of that. Maybe it was too early to see damage? I decided to speak up. "Is it normal for this to burn a lot?" I questioned the nurse.

She stopped the chemo and looked at my IV site. "Everything looks fine to me," she said as she felt my arm around the IV. She resumed the chemo but slowed down the rate.

"That still really burns," I said hesitantly.

She stopped the treatment again and re-examined my arm. At this point, both Lisa and Tracy stood up to look as well. No one saw anything.

"Some patients say that it can burn in the beginning, but then it gets better. Do you want to try again?" the nurse asked me.

I nodded. What choice did I really have? When the chemo started again, it continued to burn, but knowing that it wasn't leaking out into my tissue made me feel better. I was soon distracted by how cold my hands and feet were. The frozen mitts and socks made them painfully cold, the kind of cold I felt when I decided to go skiing in subzero temperatures with a thin pair of leather gloves (because I couldn't find my ski gloves) and crew socks (because I'd forgotten to pack my ski socks). In both instances, I envisioned my fingers and toes turning purple and falling off from frostbite.

Interestingly, my head didn't feel nearly as cold from the cold cap. *Wow, that pre-infusion cooling really works*, I thought. I assumed because the temperature of my scalp dropped slowly during the pre-infusion cycle, my scalp was spared the complete shock when the actual cooling cycle began. My hands and feet, on the other hand, were essentially plunged into the equivalent of an ice bath as soon as the mitts and socks were secured. I had to wear them for fifteen minutes, break for another fifteen, and repeat until the end of the infusion. But after five minutes, I felt like my fingertips were dying.

With my hands bound up by the mitts, I couldn't use my computer or phone to distract me, so I begged Lisa and Tracy to tell me a story.

"Oh, I have a few!" Lisa chimed. She was the queen of random stories, and for the next hour she talked about Chewie, her six-year-old shih tzu and bichon mix who looked like Chewbacca (hence his name); an upcoming trip to Spain that she was taking with her church group; her beloved Ohio State football team (Go Buckeyes!); and her annoyance with the entire electronic medical record system. Devina then popped in for a few minutes, and the four of us were finding plenty to laugh about. Before I knew it, the nurse came to disconnect the bag.

"First cycle done! Now, we're just going to run some fluids, finish the post-infusion cooling cycle, and then you're good to go." The nurse ran the fluids wide open into my IV. When the cooling system dinged to indicate that it was complete, Tracy removed the outer lining and then tried to wiggle off the inner cap.

"Ouch, stop!" I shouted. The cap had frozen to my hair, and as she tried to pull the cap off, my hair wanted to go with it. We gave it a few minutes to let it thaw and then slowly peeled it off my hair. The outer layer of my hair was frozen solid and looked like an ice helmet, but as I felt down to the scalp with my fingers, my scalp didn't feel cold at all. *That can't be good*, I thought to myself.

After we packed up all the bags, Tracy looked at me and asked, "How do you feel?"

"Great, actually." And I meant it. I felt fine. I knew I had a ton of medications running through my system, but I was surprisingly alert and energetic considering I was now going on thirty hours without sleep. "Want to go to lunch?" I suggested.

"Not exactly where I thought we'd be going after your first cycle of chemo, but why not!" Tracy smiled back.

As much anxiety as I had over chemotherapy, the actual process was pretty easy. Two different chemotherapies had been prescribed, each taking one hour to infuse. Waiting for my labs to confirm that I could get the chemo took an extra half an hour. Cold capping added another hour because of the pre-infusion and post-infusion cooling cycles. And then another hour for post-treatment hydration. A total of four and a half hours out of my life, to be repeated three more times. I totally got this.

HAIR TODAY, GONE TOMORROW

The weekend after my first cycle was surprisingly uneventful. Once I got off the steroids, my proclivity to organize and clean fell to the wayside. I spent Friday and most of Saturday sleeping and binge-watching *Love Is Blind*. Then four days after chemo, I felt well. The boys wanted to take Tracy to lunch, and she happily accepted their invitation. They insisted on an all-you-can-eat Korean BBQ restaurant, fully knowing that she and I didn't eat nearly enough to make it worth it. But it didn't matter because it was nice to have a sit-down meal with all of them. After lunch, we drove Tracy to the airport and said our goodbyes.

The following two and a half weeks were also surprisingly uneventful. While I did get a few side effects, they didn't force me to stay home or be bedbound. I considered myself fortunate to get through the first treatment relatively unscathed. I still had my hair and continued with my normal routine of work, baseball, home, and repeat, giving cancer a big middle finger and thinking, *You messed with the wrong girl. I'm not going to let you interfere with my life.*

I should have known better than to revel in how great I was doing because two weeks after the first cycle, the hair around my crown started to fall out. My bathroom floor became covered with strands of long hair, which I would gather up and throw away in a small trash can under the sink. Within three days, the trash can was full. I tried not to panic, but there seemed to be no end to how much was coming out. Eventually, my crown was completely bald, but I was able to pull back my front hair to cover this spot. *Thank God the cold capping preserved the edges of my hairline,* I thought.

And once again, I spoke too soon. Five days before my next cycle of chemo as I was sitting in bed watching TV, I ran my fingers through my hair, and my left sideburn fell out. *OMG!* I stared down at my hand looking at a clump of hair in my hand in total shock. I bolted out of bed and ran to the bathroom. I was horrified to see a huge bald spot on the left side of my head.

I dialed Tracy in a frenzy. "My . . . hair . . . is . . . falling . . . out . . ." I sobbed. She tried to calm me down, but I couldn't hear what she was saying because I was crying so hard. "This wasn't supposed to happen," I said, gasping for air.

Up until this point, I didn't look like a cancer patient. No one could tell I'd had mastectomies, and no one could tell that I was getting chemo. But with a chunk of my hair missing from the side of my head, it would be obvious that something was going on. And without hair, I looked sick. I didn't want to look sick because I didn't want to be treated differently. I didn't want people's sympathy. I wanted to be treated normally, but I'd never be treated normally if I didn't look normal. *This wasn't supposed to happen,* I kept repeating to myself.

"Are you still there?" Tracy asked.

"I need to call my sister. My family is supposed to come here next weekend for Easter, and I don't want them to see me without my hair. I need to tell them not to come. I haven't told my dad. He will freak out if I don't have hair." I started crying again.

I dialed Min. When she picked up, I was too choked up to talk.

"Sue, what's wrong?" she asked with a slight panic to her voice.

"My hair. It's falling out."

"It'll be okay," she tried to reassure me.

"I don't want you coming next weekend. I don't want any of you to see me like this."

Then Min started to break down on the other line. "We haven't seen you since your diagnosis. We need to come, Sue. We want to be there to support you. We want to see you. Please don't cancel the trip."

"I may have no hair!" I screamed. "How are we supposed to explain that to Dad? Remember Dad, the guy we decided not to tell?"

"Dad is half blind!" she laughed back. "He can barely see out of one eye." And she was right for the most part. Our dad had struggled with glaucoma for as long as I could remember, which severely affected his visual acuity as he got older.

"Fine," I sniffled back. "I won't cancel the trip. Bye."

"Sue!" Devina hollered as she shut the front door behind her. "Where are you?" She wandered into my bedroom and found me sitting in my recliner.

"So this just happened," I said as I held up my left sideburn.

"I know. Tracy called me and told me to get over here." She took my sideburn from me and held it up to her ponytail. "Are you aware you have more hair in your sideburn than I do in my ponytail?"

I tried to laugh, but I was devastated. I knew my hair would grow back, but the cancer had already taken my breasts. Why couldn't it just leave my hair alone? Over the years, my hair had become a big part of my identity. It's what people always noticed about me. It's what people envied about me. And it's what made me feel feminine.

Up until the age of ten, I was forced to sport a bowl cut, so people always confused me for a boy. Add neutral-colored clothing and it's understandable why I spent much of my childhood being called a he instead of a she. Although I was allowed to grow my hair longer once I entered middle school, being called a boy left an indelible impact on how I saw myself as I entered the volatile teenage and young adult years. My hair was about so much more than just vanity, it was a significant part of my identity.

I felt this disease slowly stripping meaningful parts of me away, which was an aspect of cancer care that I overlooked when counseling patients. I often wondered, *Why are we crying over breasts and hair when we are dealing with cancer?* I then thought of my newly diagnosed patients who wanted both their breasts removed yesterday, even if they were excellent candidates for breast preservation. And I wondered if these patients were prepared for the impact it would have on their body image and self-esteem.

"We will get you a nice lace wig. Let's go tomorrow to look," she suggested.

"What's a lace wig?" I asked.

"Oh, lots of people have them! You just don't know it because it looks natural." Devina pulled up some pictures on her phone, and I was surprised and impressed by what I saw. "You've never had to think much about this, Sue, because you have great hair. But most women don't, so they have to rely on hair extensions, toppers, and wigs to get the hair they want."

And she was right. When I looked up the stats, about half of American women wear wigs or hair extensions. Suddenly, something that was totally abnormal to me wasn't so abnormal.

The next morning, I stepped in the shower before going wig shopping. As soon as I started shampooing my hair, all the loose strands got caught up in my fingers. I picked them out one by one and let them fall to the floor. As I gently ran my fingers through my hair, more fell out. After a few minutes, the shower drain was clogged, and water started to rise to my ankles. Every expletive ran through my mind as I looked at clumps of hair floating in the shallow pool of water that I was now standing in. I began rinsing the shampoo out, but this caused huge balls of loose hair to get tangled in the hair that hadn't fallen out. I tried my best to untangle everything, but my efforts just made the hair balls grow bigger and bigger. I then grabbed the conditioner and liberally coated everything, thinking that would detangle the nest that was now forming on my head, but it didn't help at all. Nothing helped. Not knowing what to do, I got out of the shower dripping wet and called Devina.

"I need help," I pleaded as I looked at the knotty mess that my hair had become.

"Put some clothes on and come over," she directed me.

Within fifteen minutes, I was walking through her front door. "Hello? Anyone home?"

"In here!" she yelled back. When I walked into the master bathroom, she was standing there with Andrea and Alicja, who had set up a mini salon. There was a chair in the middle of the bathroom, with large and fine-tooth combs, several detangling sprays, and (worst case scenario) scissors lined up neatly on the counter. They all slowly worked together to extract the hair balls while preserving the hair that was still holding on for dear life. Alicja worked on the left side of my head, Andrea the right, and Devina took the front. After an hour, all but one knot had been removed. They combined their efforts to conquer the last knot, but I could tell it was so entangled that scissors would be required. None of them wanted to admit it. They just kept working together pulling each strand of hair out one by one. I deeply admired their perseverance and was touched by their dedication but finally called off the rescue efforts.

"Get the scissors."

I heard a collective sigh of relief as they threw their combs down on the counter and stretched their overworked fingers. None of them wanted to pick up the scissors and make the final cut. Because the knot was so high up, it would be impossible to preserve any length to that section of hair. Finally, Alicja spoke up in her commanding Polish accent, "Devina, you are the surgeon. You do it." Andrea handed her the scissors like a scrub nurse handing over a scalpel. She reluctantly took them and methodically snipped away, and we watched more hair fall to the ground. We fell silent, as if we were at a funeral for my hair that didn't survive the first round of chemo, transfixed by the mess on the floor.

I turned to look at the mirror and said nothing as I stared at my reflection. I still had long hair over the front part of my scalp, but I was sideburnless and only had a thin layer of hair remaining on the sides. I could use the intact hair to cover the bald spot on my crown or the sparse areas on the sides, but not both. It was a strange experience to sit there with my closest friends and watch my former "healthy" self fade into a balding cancer patient.

"Thanks for the memories," I lamented. "Let's go wig shopping." We quickly cleaned the hair from the floor and headed downtown to the stores where the drag queens shopped. They always had the best wigs.

GOING PUBLIC

On the first Sunday night following my initial chemo treatment, I experienced a sudden onset of horrific bone pain, which I knew was from Neulasta, a drug that stimulates white blood cell production. While I had pre-medicated with Claritin, a medication commonly used for allergies but also proven to be effective for alleviating bone pain, it didn't help. I lay still in the recliner, at times wondering if the pain in my chest bone was what a heart attack felt like. Not wanting to cry because the boys were nearby, I focused on taking deep breaths through the discomfort. Shifting my focus to breathwork took my mind off the pain and helped me eventually fall asleep. The next morning, I called Wassim to yell at him. I knew it wasn't his fault, but it just felt good to yell at someone—anyone. Once he saw that my post-chemo counts were good, he reduced the dose of Neulasta, which effectively took away the pain with the subsequent injections. Patients would often tell me how debilitating the bone pain from Neulasta was, and now I knew firsthand exactly what they meant.

Once the bone pain resolved, I developed an annoying upper eyelid twitch, the kind I would experience when I got tired from reading too much. The kind that causes people to look at you curiously as it's happening. The kind where the more you focus on it, the longer it lasts. When I asked Wassim, he said it was stress related. When I asked the internet, Dr. Google informed me that it could be due to Taxotere affecting the nerves of the eyelid. Dr. Google also said it would resolve by itself.

Around the same time of the twitching, I also developed a large bruise on the entire backside of my left forearm. When I was in the breast clinic seeing patients, Vickie, one of Wassim's nurses, commented on my "impressive thrombophlebitis." "Nothing to be concerned about, Doc. The vein just got really irritated from the chemo. At least the chemo didn't extravasate," she informed me. "The discoloration will go away with time."

The last side effect I experienced, which was totally unexpected, was an incredibly itchy rash on the back of my thighs, groin, neck, and armpits. The itching was so severe, even with steroid cream, that I clawed off the top layer of skin in several spots. It was worse in heat, which made it challenging since my boys were in tournaments every weekend in the hot Florida sun. If I couldn't get a parking spot by the outfield to cheer them on from the comfort of my air-conditioned car, I would set up camp under a beach umbrella, with a portable fan, lots of cold water, and a layer of white steroid cream applied to my legs, neck, and arm. I could only imagine how amazing I looked, with straggly hair that was partially covered by my baseball cap, an eye that twitched uncontrollably, a large bruise on my forearm, and white cream covering my legs, neck, and arms. But I didn't care because I was there to support my kids. If people stared too long, I would raise my forearm so they could get a better look and joke, "I promise I'm not contagious."

Much to my surprise, my kids weren't phased by my new look. I initially used them as the major reason I needed to preserve my hair. "It will be too much of a shock for them. I don't want them to be traumatized by this experience," I explained to others. But as my hair fell out, they didn't have any anxiety or panic, and I credited Devina with this because she talked to them quite a bit about what to expect. One day James said to me, "Uh Mom . . . what look are you going for exactly? You think it's time to buzz it all off?"

Once I realized they didn't care, I attempted to shave it off... several times. I would call Devina in the morning and tell her,

"Ok, I'm ready. I'll be over after work." And then I would chicken out at the end of the day and call her to cancel.

The last time I cancelled, I did manage to make it over to her house. I had just finished playing tennis with Dave, an incredibly energetic friend who was always looking for the next good commercial real estate deal, a good time, or both. He had an extensive network of friends, acquaintances, and business connections and was a walking version of LinkedIn, gladly making connections every chance he got. He also understood my sons' baseball lives since he hailed from baseball royalty—his great grandfather was Ty Cobb. We met through our tennis coach, Danny, who wanted him to practice with better players. At the time, I was hesitant knowing that there would be a big difference in our playing abilities. But he was also a college basketball player, so I figured he would be naturally athletic and have a competitive drive to get better. We eventually became mixed doubles partners and close friends—treating each other like siblings and creating a pact with one another that whoever we might be dating had to accept us as a pair, otherwise that person had to go.

After we finished tennis, I felt a sudden urge to shave off my hair.

"Let's do it!" Dave exclaimed. "I'll record it for you."

We ended up at Devina's house a few minutes later and I was back in the bathroom where my friends once worked tirelessly to preserve the hair that I now wanted to get rid of.

"You okay?" Dave asked cautiously.

"I look ridiculous. And my kids don't care." I stared in the mirror, shocked at what remained. From the front, I still saw my old self. From the back, I was essentially bald with a small chunk of hair at the base of my skull that I affectionately called my rat tail.

Devina plugged in the clippers and turned them on. I could hear the loud buzzing next to my ear. Dave pulled out his phone and took a pre-shave video. He then moved next to Devina, who looked me directly in the eyes and nervously asked, "Ready?"

"Uh, hold on." I looked at my reflection in the mirror one more time and caught a glimpse of my precancer self. I then thought of all the times my patients said shaving their heads gave them a strong sense of control over their cancer—they weren't going to let the chemo make them bald; they would do it themselves. I also remembered others who'd shaved because they hated watching their hair continuously fall out. Whenever anyone asked my professional opinion, I favored shaving so they could have a fresh start. And now here I was, looking at myself in the mirror thinking what a hypocrite I was, unable to do the very thing that I had recommended others to do.

"Put away the clippers. I can't do this."

I was done trying to shave my head. Who was I kidding? I would never be ready to take it all off because the remaining hair represented my precancer self, a person who took for granted her health, assumed she would always be around for her kids, and had no fear of imminent death. While that life was by no means stress free, it held the promise of unlimited potential because there would always be a tomorrow. I never fully appreciated the luxury of looking at life through these rose-colored glasses until cancer smashed them into little pieces.

Ever since I was a young child, I've always been about delayed gratification. "Work hard now so that you can do whatever you want in the future," my parents constantly reminded me. In high school, I studied hard and wasn't allowed to party. Once I got into a good college, I studied harder and partied a little. Then while I was in medical school, my college friends got jobs in the real world and enjoyed their young adulthood. Then I went to residency, where I continued my education, got married, and gave birth to my first child. After training, I started working as an attending and during this period of my life, I had two more children, built my medical practice, and saved for retirement, when I would finally be able to explore things that interested me, travel, and do whatever I wanted.

I know it must sound odd to wait until retirement to "find myself," but I learned how commonplace this was as I spent more time talking to my patients. One patient in particular stood out for me. She was a seventy-five-year-old woman who was four years out from treatment.

"I need you to get more exercise. Go for a walk, thirty minutes, five times a week," I advised.

"I can walk, but it's boring," she replied.

"Do you play any sports? Have any outdoor hobbies that you enjoy doing?" I questioned.

"No, I don't. Honestly, Doc, I sit at home and watch TV because I don't know what I like to do." She paused for a minute. "I've spent my life taking care of others. I have no idea what I like. First, I took care of my siblings when I was younger, then my own children, then my husband when he fell ill, and then my mother, who died two months ago. Now I have no one to take care of."

As I listened to her, I felt like I was kind of living her life—always taking care of someone in my adult life. If it weren't for tennis, which I had only recently picked up again after a twenty year hiatus, I could be her. Outside of work, the boys, and their activities, I didn't really have much time to explore what I truly enjoyed.

"Well," I looked at her and smiled, "there is no time like the present. Seminole County has a great recreational program guide.

Maybe look through the brochure and try a few things. You won't know until you try. You've spent so much time putting others before you. Now is your time. I am writing you a prescription to find a hobby." Then I took out my prescription pad, scribbled a few words, tore off the paper, and handed it to her. "I want to see you back in six months with an update."

I'd never used my prescription pad to dispense anything other than medication but felt that this one prescription was just as impactful as any medication I could have prescribed. Before my diagnosis, my typical follow-up entailed performing breast exams, reviewing surveillance imaging and labs, and determining if the radiation caused any long-term issues with the breast. Cancer control was my priority, while addressing other issues took a backseat. Once I became a patient however, it was impossible to continue practicing this way because now, I was part of this sisterhood. And even though it was a sisterhood that no one ever wants to be in, in this sisterhood, we all look out for one another, encourage one another, and push one other to be healthier, happier, and more fulfilled.

"I was looking forward to seeing what cute outfit you were going to wear today," she said as I walked her back to the waiting room.

"Oh, I had to go to the OR today," I lied. The truth was I'd stopped wearing dresses to the office because the easiest way to conceal my hair loss was with a scrub cap. But with the scrub cap came scrubs, and no one was the wiser. While our cancer center had a wonderful wig specialist who made a wig that looked exactly like my hair, the wig was itchy and uncomfortable to wear. I was so preoccupied that it was lopsided or about to fall off that I was unable to focus on anything else. So as great as wigs were in theory, I didn't find it practical and quickly abandoned it for scrub caps.

"Can I give you a hug?" she asked.

I nodded. As we embraced, she whispered in my ear, "A mutual acquaintance told me about your diagnosis. I want you to know I'm so sorry that you have to deal with this, but now I know you understand me."

As I drove home that evening, I kept thinking about what my patient had said to me. *I* truly got her, and she was right. It's not that I didn't have an understanding as the doctor, but it was different now that I was the one sitting on the exam table. I knew lots of doctors got cancer, and I knew that lots of oncologists got cancer, but it was a unique experience to get the cancer that I specialized in and to receive multimodality treatment—mastectomy, reconstruction, chemotherapy, radiation, targeted therapy, and endocrine therapy—all while continuing to treat the disease in others. *To treat while being treated.*

When I first found out I had cancer, I asked why a lot because if I understood the why, I thought it would make it easier to come to terms with the diagnosis. But now I found myself asking why because the why would help me better understand my purpose. I do believe everything happens for a reason. And that patient made me realize my diagnosis offered me a deeper connection with those I treat, a connection that wasn't possible as a spectator and a connection that renewed my desire to be an even better advocate for my patients. For the first time since hearing that I had five masses in my breast, I was beginning to see the value of sharing my breast cancer with others. In some strange way, letting others know helped me come to terms with my own new reality. The more I told others, the more I couldn't deny it anymore.

But letting others in would also remind them of how non-discriminatory breast cancer could be. Many friends commented on the irony of a breast cancer doctor getting breast cancer, but in reality, it affects one in every eight women. So why was it so ironic? My diagnosis prompted an open discussion on breast cancer screening, especially for those who have never gone or for those who were overdue. If the "irony" of my diagnosis would help more women go for their mammograms, then I would willingly share what had happened. I also realized that by sharing my story, I could show them that I had gotten through it and so could they. I finally found a deeper purpose through my diagnosis.

When I got home, I headed to my bathroom to get changed. As I looked at myself in the mirror with my scrub cab on, I looked no different than before my diagnosis. But as soon as I took the cap off, the reality of my situation was evident. While I'm not one to be known for selfies, I set my camera up and recorded myself removing the scrub cap. I undid the long strands of hair from the bobby pins that held them up, exposing my thinned-out hair and balding crown. Once the recording was finished, I sat in my bed and started typing my thoughts. Before I knew it, I had made a reel. I didn't share it; I kept it to myself. But it felt good to honestly express myself.

The reel sat for days in my drafts. I wasn't quite sure what to do with it. I was never very big on social media. I used it to keep tabs on others but rarely shared my own life on it. I knew something needed to change. I couldn't keep pretending everything was normal while looking like I was going to the OR all the time. Maybe it was time to own my story.

Purpose through diagnosis. I started an Instagram page @ breast_cancer_360—a name that reflected the doctor and patient perspective I now had on the disease. I was terrified, but I kept thinking of my favorite quote that I'd heard on NPR just that morning, "Comfort is the enemy of growth." I had to get a little uncomfortable to grow, so I worked up the courage and finally hit post. As a doctor, I was used to being the one with answers. Now, as a patient, I was about to publicly acknowledge how many questions and uncertainties I still had.

The response was overwhelming. Messages flooded in—from patients, from other doctors, from friends, and strangers facing their own battles. "Thank you for sharing this," they wrote. "Thank you for being real about it." So many people reminded me that they were there for me and the boys if I needed. I felt so loved.

Eventually, each post became a little easier, and each share felt a little more natural. I wasn't just Dr. Hwang anymore, dispensing medical wisdom from behind a professional persona. I was also Sue, figuring this out one day at a time, just like everyone else. The hair loss, too, became part of the story—not the whole story but a chapter in it. The wigs became props in a larger narrative about vulnerability, strength, and the messy space between the two. And somewhere along the way, I stopped trying to maintain the perfect image of a doctor going through cancer and started being a person going through cancer treatment who happened to be a doctor. This was becoming the journey I needed to share.

THE EMOTIONAL TSUNAMI

I've had many patients talk about the emotional roller coaster of endocrine therapy. It's especially hard on those who are pre-menopausal at the time of diagnosis. I personally have never been a particularly emotional person, and thought I'd be immune to this aspect of estrogen deprivation since I'd received Lupron shortly after my surgery and felt no difference.

Then came the sudden onset of emotional swings like I'd never experienced before. One morning, after dropping Nathan off at school, I started crying. I didn't know why I was crying, but I was . . . uncontrollably. My closest friend from medical school, Margaret, had the unfortunate luck of calling me at this moment. I answered the phone sobbing.

"What's wrong?" she asked with a concerned tone.

"I don't know. I'm just sad. I can't explain it," I managed to say between gasps for air.

"You're going through *so* much right now, Sue. I don't know how you handle it." She didn't know what else to say. But she stayed on the line, silent, as I continued crying. Even though she wasn't saying anything, just knowing she was there brought me comfort. I met Margaret on my first day of medical school. I didn't know anyone, whereas she knew half the class, having gone to Northwestern for undergrad. She had called out to her friend, Susan, who was walking in front of me, but I turned around. And without missing a beat, she started talking to me as if I was the person she intended to speak to. That incident pretty much describes Margaret to a tee—never wanting to make anyone feel bad and always accommodating in any situation.

"Do you need me to come down?" she asked, even though she had three kids of her own and was one of the busiest ophthalmologists in Atlanta.

"You are an amazing friend, but no. I just have to get used to this no estrogen thing. You caught me at a bad time. I'm sorry for being such a mess."

"I love you, Sue. I'm here if you need me." I knew she meant it. She would drop everything to be by my side if I needed her.

"I'm good. I just parked. I need to go to work. Love you too," I said sniffling.

As I walked to my office, I looked to see if Wassim was in but his office was empty. I wasn't sad, exactly. I wasn't angry, either. I was just . . . overwhelmed. Everything felt too much—the weight of being both doctor and patient, parenting, the physical demands of recovery, and now the chemotherapy.

I got to my office and shut the door. I started sobbing again. I couldn't control it. It was like the floodgates opened wide and all these emotions I didn't know I had came spilling out.

"Doc," I heard Marie say on the other side of my door. I didn't respond, but she could hear me crying, so she opened the door and quickly closed it behind her. "What can I do?" she asked as she gave me a big hug.

I couldn't say anything. I just kept sobbing. She handed me the box of tissues that was sitting at the edge of my desk.

"I'll be right back." She left my office, and a few minutes later, she came back with Wassim.

"Sue?" Wassim asked as he knelt beside my office chair.

"I can't stop crying." I started heaving at this point.

"This isn't you," he reassured me. "You have no more estrogen, and your body is in shock."

I couldn't talk. I managed to stop crying, but if I tried to talk, I would start crying again.

"Do you want me to prescribe Effexor?" he asked.

"No!" Effexor is an antidepressant that's commonly prescribed to breast cancer patients because it helps manage emotional lability as well as hot flashes. I encouraged women to go on it all the time, but I didn't want to be on it myself. *I* was fine. *I* didn't have any issues that needed medication.

"It will help with the hot flashes too," he explained.

"I don't want it. I don't need it." I continued to sob. I was beyond the point of reasoning at this point, so he dropped the subject.

"You will feel better. I promise." He gave me another hug.

"Doc, I'm going to see if Dr. Stall can see the first few patients in the morning for you. You aren't in any condition to be seeing patients right now." Marie and Wassim left my office together, closing the door behind them.

Get a grip, I kept telling myself. *Why are you crying? There's no reason to be crying!*

There was another knock at my door. "Sue?" I heard Bronwyn call softly from the other side. "Marie told me what's going on. I'm going to see your first few patients. I can see more if you need. Just let me know." And then she was gone. Bronwyn was one of my partners and someone that I really liked as a person even though I didn't know her very well. She was a hard-working physician who spent as much time with her patients as they needed. She emanated kindness and compassion and had a calming energy about her. She was also the mother to three boys and understood the struggles of being a physician mom.

Eventually, I was able to collect myself and carried on with the rest of my day as if nothing had happened. As I left the office at the end of the day and headed to my car, my mentor, E, called me.

"Just checking in," she said casually. She was another boss lady whom I admired. I had met her when I rotated through the emergency department at Northwestern. After just graduating from medical school, I developed a sudden mental block when I was assigned my first patient as a doctor. She was a senior surgical resident finishing up a consult and saw the panic on my face. Even though she had no idea who I was, she pulled me aside and said, "You wouldn't be working at one of the best hospitals in the country if you didn't know your stuff. Take a deep breath, go in that room and do your thing." Whatever anxiety I had was wiped out by the authority in her voice. I thanked her and she gave me her number in case I ever needed another motivational talk. We kept in close contact even after she left Northwestern and established herself as a preeminent surgeon in the Midwest. I commonly called her for advice about how to navigate the complex world of medicine. When I heard her voice over the phone, my floodgates reopened.

"Is it the Lupron?" she questioned.

"It is," I admitted. "My medical oncologist wants me to go on Effexor, but I said no."

"Why?"

"I don't want to be on it. I know I tell patients to be on it all the time, but I don't want to be on it." It was a crappy explanation, but it was all I had.

"I think you need it. I don't know how you are doing it. Cancer, chemo, kids, work. There's only so much you can juggle at one time." E paused for a moment. "Sue, it's not a sign of weakness. It's a sign of strength."

I didn't know what to say in response. I wasn't sure where she was going with the conversation.

"Do you remember right after Little E passed?" she asked.

"How could I forget?" And it was true. How could I ever forget that time? E had been happily married since medical school, but beyond being a successful surgeon, she always wanted to be a mother. But the first four times she got pregnant, she miscarried toward the end of the first trimester. Until Little E. E didn't tell anyone about the pregnancy until she made it to the third trimester, and when she announced that she and her husband were expecting a little girl soon, her closest friends came together from across the country to throw a surprise baby shower six weeks before her due date. She was radiant. And then a week later, her husband called to tell me that the baby stopped moving. Little E was gone.

"I never told you this, but after we buried Little E, I was driving home along this winding road, and I thought to myself, *What if I just keep this wheel straight and go off the cliff? I could see Little E again.* I missed her so much. I wanted to be with her so much. I saw my future with her, and without her, I couldn't see a future anymore."

I didn't know what to say. I knew the loss of Little E was devastating but never knew her pain was so great that she considered suicide.

"I almost went off the road, Sue. I would have been happy to drive off the road. But I didn't. I thought of my husband. He had been through just as much pain as I had, but he was still here. How could I leave him?" She paused for a minute. "The next day, I started Paxil. I needed it for that point in my life. I didn't need it forever, but I needed it then."

"I never knew. I'm so sorry."

"Not many people know this about me, but I'm telling you because I think you need Effexor for right now. Until things get better, it will help you adapt. It's not a sign of weakness. Your body can only deal with so much, and at some point, you will crack. The medication stabilizes the crack until your body is ready to mend it. It's not a sign of weakness, I promise," she repeated.

As E spoke, my mind raced: *My brilliant friend and a highly respected doctor had these thoughts? What?*

"Go on Effexor," she advised. "There's nothing wrong with it. This is just too much for you to handle alone."

Coming from E—practical, no-nonsense E—this message hit home. I felt as if I'd been given permission to be human, to need help, and to not have to be strong all the time. This was exactly what I needed to hear, even if I didn't know it until that moment.

The hormonal upheaval wasn't just emotional—it manifested physically too. Hot flashes began ambushing me at random moments. Sleep became elusive. My body felt like it was at war with itself, and in many ways, it was. The treatment that was supposed to save my life was making that life feel increasingly unmanageable. Yet somehow, I had to find a way forward.

E was right. I needed help. It was time I accepted that. And more importantly, it was okay to take it. After a few weeks of taking the medication, I could feel the improvement. It was as if the Effexor acted like a thermostat for my emotions, turning up the heat when the "lows" hit and nudging me back toward balance. I still experienced moments of sadness, but there were just that—moments, passing almost as quickly as they came.

RINGING THE BELL

The last day of chemotherapy finally arrived. "Time to ring the bell," the nurse announced cheerfully as she removed my IV. I didn't really want to ring the bell because radiation still loomed ahead. But as Tracy, Lisa, and I made our way to the front desk of the infusion center, all the nurses and front desk staff gathered to cheer me on. *Well*, I thought, *when in Rome . . .*

I stared at the brass bell mounted on the wall. The faces of my patients who had done this before me flashed before my eyes, and now it was my time. So, I grabbed the rope and rang the heck out of it.

"Uh, Doc?" the nurse interrupted as she pointed to the plaque by the side of the bell.

I let go of the rope and read the poem engraved in the plaque. "Ring this bell / Three times well / It's toll to clearly say / My treatment's done / This course is run / And I am on my way!" *Oooops*, I thought to myself. *Only three times.*

"Redo?" I asked as I looked at the nurse.

She nodded with a smile.

I rang the bell three times. Lisa, Tracy, and I took some pictures with the chemo nurses. I got my certificate, and we headed to my car.

"Don't hate me, okay?" Tracy said. "Just one more stop."

I had no idea what she was talking about until we ended up at my office.

"One more bell. I know this is the radiation bell, but everyone wanted to be here to support the end of your chemo. It's supposed to be a surprise, so look surprised," she instructed as we got out of the car.

I walked through the patient entrance and saw Devina, Wassim, our entire office staff, and the hospital administration standing there clapping. I was overwhelmed and thankful for the Effexor, otherwise I would have burst out crying seeing everyone there in celebration of my last day of chemo. I walked over to the bell, read the poem aloud, and rang the bell exactly three times. *Three times.* No more, no less. Even this celebration had its protocols.

The first ring was for my kids—for Nathan's worried questions, for Sam's quiet presence, for James's need for the facts.

The second ring was for my team—for Tracy's middle-of-the-night support, for Devina's unwavering presence, for Lisa coming out of retirement to operate on me, for Wassim putting up with my rants, and for all the staff that had become my supportive family.

The third ring . . . I hesitated. The third ring was supposed to be for me, but who was I now? Not just a doctor anymore. Not just a patient. Not just a mother. Something new, something changed, something still emerging from this transformative chrysalis of treatment.

I rang it anyway.

The room erupted in applause—everyone celebrating this moment.

After all the pictures were taken and hugs were given, I looked back at that bell. How many times had I told patients, "You'll get here someday"? Now I understood both the truth and the complexity of that promise. You get here, yes, but you're different from when you arrived.

SLEEPING BEAUTY

After the last cycle of chemo was completed and the bells were run, I got my first taste of truly debilitating fatigue. Up until this point, I spent the first few days after chemo resting, going between the living room couch, my recliner, and my bed. I was tired but still able to engage with the boys, who met me where I was at. Movie nights happened in my room, with kids sprawled across my bed while I dozed in and out. Conversations moved to wherever I had the energy to be. And sometimes, they would lay down next to me and say nothing. It wasn't ideal by any means, but I was still able to be there for them.

The last cycle however was different. The exhaustion hit me like a tidal wave, a bone-deep kind of exhaustion that made getting out of bed feel like climbing Everest. Two days after the last cycle, I didn't even have enough energy to watch TV. I shut the blinds in my bedroom and slept for the next thirty-six hours.

"Are you going to die?" Nathan asked when I made no effort to get out of my bed. It reminded me of when I first told him of my diagnosis. But now the question had more weight, more context. He'd seen me weak. He'd seen me human.

"I'm just really tired, buddy," I mumbled as I dozed off to sleep again. Amazingly, the boys adapted. They found ways to be close to me without needing me. Every few hours, Sam would come in to hug me and kiss me on the cheek. Before leaving the room, he'd ask if I needed anything and inform me he did his homework. James gave me detailed updates on baseball, filling the silence with stories that required no response from me. And Nathan just crawled into my bed and watched movies as I slept.

The house was different that weekend. For the two days that I slept away, it was eerily quiet. There was no fighting. The typical chaos of three boys under one roof disappeared. No one was making fun of anyone. No one was asking me where something was. No one yelled, "Mom!" Even the dogs seemed to understand the mood as they stood guard by my bed.

In those moments of forced stillness, something unexpected happened. My kids learned to be caregivers while still being kids. They learned that strength sometimes looks like asking for help, that love sometimes looks like sitting quietly beside someone who's suffering, that family sometimes means just being there, even when there's nothing you can do to fix what's broken.

Chapter Seven
TREATING AND BEING TREATED

"Please add Ms. Wilson to the schedule today," I said to Marie, who turned to her computer to see where we could fit her in.

"Only thing we have is at the end of the day. Tell her 5:00 PM," she reported back while typing the patient's information into the computer.

"That won't work. She doesn't drive and relies on her daughter for transportation. Her daughter has to be at work by 2:00 PM," I explained.

"Well, unless someone cancels, we will have to treat her tomorrow."

"But she's in a lot of pain." I moved behind Marie to look at the schedule. We have two treatment machines at our facility, and both were packed back-to-back with patients until the end of the day. There really was no room to add anyone new except for the end of the day. "Give her some of my time. I won't need the forty-five minutes that were blocked for my start. I know this will be my first treatment, but I know the drill. Put her in at noon, and then you can slip me in right after. Or you can just put me in at the end of the day. It's not like I won't be here." Certainly not the most ideal way to start my first day of radiation, but I foresaw my treatment as being uncomplicated. I had, after all, supervised thousands of treatments and knew exactly what to expect. I wouldn't have new patient jitters or need the new patient orientation talk that took the therapists five minutes to deliver.

Marie looked at me with uncertainty, caught between respecting me as her doctor and treating me as a patient. It was a dance we were all learning—this awkward choreography of shifting power dynamics. I knew exactly how our schedule worked, but now that I was on the other side of it, I was just another patient needing to be fitted into the day's workflow.

"Dr. Hwang, it's your first treatment today. You really should have the fully allocated time in case . . . ," she started, then stopped, clearly unsure whether to push back against my suggestion.

I understood her hesitation. After all, I was still technically her boss. But I was also her patient, and she was right. While the patient in me didn't want anyone rushing because we were short on time, the doctor in me wanted to accommodate my patient who was in pain.

"I agree with you," I acknowledged. "But she needs to be treated." And our discussion was over.

When Ms. Wilson's daughter wheelchaired her into my office, I knew I'd made the right decision. I could tell she was in a lot of pain by the way she was awkwardly sitting in the chair. Brittany, one of the radiation therapists, wheeled her back to the treatment room. After the patient was set up on the treatment table, the therapists stepped out to take verification X-rays. Despite the pain, she was perfectly positioned on the table, and I okayed the treatment to begin. As the machine delivered the radiation, I looked at the live video of her on the table and thought, *That could be me right now . . . That will be me next. My turn soon.*

Once treatment was complete, I sat in the control room as the therapists entered the vault to help Ms. Wilson back into her wheelchair. As she passed me on the way out, she grabbed my arm and said, "Thank you. My daughter said there were no times today, but you made it happen. God bless."

"Ready?" Brittany asked as she returned from the waiting room and headed into the vault to prep the room. I stood behind her, not knowing whether to help her or whether to get changed. For the first time since my first day of residency, I didn't know my place in the treatment room.

"You are the patient now," Marie informed me as she walked in. "Get changed and put on the gown. We'll be ready for you in a minute."

Thank God for Marie, I thought to myself. As the therapist manager, she was used to commanding people around, even the doctor. The other therapists, I could sense, were nervous. While they had treated friends and acquaintances previously, they had never treated a breast radiation oncologist who they knew was OCD about every little detail. Even though Bronwyn was the supervising doctor, they knew I'd be reviewing what they did after the fact. I totally understood the awkwardness of this situation. I also couldn't imagine getting treated anywhere else because I felt comfort in being treated by the therapists that I trained. We had so much history together and they knew how I thought. In addition, getting treatment at my own center allowed me to continue working without having to take time off to go elsewhere.

"On the table, Doc," Marie instructed as she patted the table with her hand. My staff was patient and professional, treating me just like any other patient. But I could feel the weight of their eyes, the careful way they gave instructions to someone who usually gave them orders.

As I sat on the table, I started getting nervous. All the concerns that my patients had about radiation, that I would gently reassure them were not likely to happen, came flooding into my mind. Pain. Chest wall tightness. Capsular contraction. Radiation-induced cancer. The last one lingered on my mind. It was always the complication that I spent the most time reviewing with patients even though it was the one that was least likely to happen.

"What do you mean radiation can cause cancer? I *have* cancer. Why would I do a treatment that would give me another cancer?" patients would always ask me. And I would always give the same reply. "Nothing in medicine is without risk, but then again nothing in life is either. Your risk of dying in a car accident in the US is higher than your risk of getting a cancer from radiation, but you still get in a car every day of your life." Reframing the risk always helped patients feel more comfortable with treatment; however, all I could think about as I got on the table were my patients that had developed cancers from treatment. Sure, I could count the number of those patients on one hand (compared to the thousands of women that I've treated), but it's really different telling someone the statistics versus living the possibility of the statistics.

The irony wasn't lost on me. A radiation oncologist getting a radiation-induced cancer—the treatment that I prescribed to so many, the treatment that I made my livelihood on, the treatment that allowed me to afford a comfortable lifestyle for my family, was also the same treatment that *could* lead to my own demise. Chances were slim . . . but then again so were the chances of a breast radiation oncologist getting breast cancer and needing radiation. I ran through the numbers in my head. 340 million people in the US, out of which 140 million are women, out of which only 1,590 are radiation oncologists, out of which 198 will get breast cancer, out of which 99 will need radiation. The chances of getting cancer from radiation were much greater than the chances of being a radiation oncologist who gets breast cancer and needs radiation.

I laid down on the treatment table and into the mold of my upper torso and upper arms that was created during my planning session. The mold was hard and cold but absolutely necessary to ensure that I was in the same exact position every day for treatment. As Brittany and Marie worked to place my body in perfect alignment, I looked at the ceiling of the treatment room. It was the standard foam panels that were typical in hospitals and office buildings. I'd never noticed the little divots in the panels before. Come to think of it, I don't think I ever really looked at the ceiling of the treatment room, but then again why would I? Funny how you discover new things about a room when you're forced to lie still and stare upward. Had all my patients noticed these same spots? Had they created their own stories about the patterns in the tiles?

Then I studied the head of the linear accelerator, which was the machine that generates the high energy X-rays that treat cancer, as it stared me right in the face. I counted the number of nuts and bolts to pass time. They were so small but so critical to the integrity of the machine, and without them everything would fall apart. But they were never what patients asked about when evaluating the quality of the equipment. They were overlooked in terms of importance, but they reminded me that it's the small things in life that matter.

"Your setup looks great. We are going to step out of the room and take some pictures." I heard them hit the button on the wall that triggered the heavy lead door to close. I was alone in the room, holding perfectly still. My eyes darted around the dimly lit room. My attention was drawn to a rack that held all my patients' molds—molds that I had made countless times before but never noticed just how hard and how cold they were until I lay in mine. I saw the chair that patients would sit in as I explained potential complications. I noticed the box of tissues on the side table that I handed to scared patients who were doing their best to hold it all in. Things that were so mundane when I was the physician were now keeping me mentally occupied as I waited for the treatment to start.

The machine started to rotate around me, capturing images of my breast and chest. Because radiation can't be seen or felt, the machine produces a beeping sound to let the patient know the beam was on. *Beep . . . beep . . . beep . . . beep . . . beep . . .* The beeping seemed never ending as the machine spun around my body. Finally, it stopped. *Okay,* I thought to myself, *we should be ready to start in a few minutes.* Those minutes went by, and then a few more minutes went by. I was running through the possibilities for why it was taking so long. Bronwyn was in the control room when I got on the table, so I knew they weren't waiting for the doctor. This must have meant that there was something wrong with my setup and that they were trying to figure out what adjustment to make, but even if that were true, it shouldn't have taken this long. Then I thought they must have had to call a physicist to either override a parameter or get their okay on the images. But that didn't happen often. What was making my setup so complex that they needed a physicist? *Say something,* I thought to myself. *It's okay to ask what is going on. But if I ask what's going on, Bronwyn will be offended and annoyed. Don't be that patient, Sue. We all know what the staff thinks of those patients.* I kept my mouth shut and waited. Suddenly, Brittany Spears came on overhead. I could almost feel the vibrations of the opening beats.

"Everything looks good," Marie said. "Here's your first treatment."

Here we go. Hit me, baby, one more time.

RADIATION REALITIES

A radiation therapy schedule becomes its own kind of time-keeper. Ideally, every patient is given a schedule at the start of treatment, so they know how to plan the days out. And the schedule typically blocks the same time every day for the patient to keep things consistent. If every patient under treatment had a different time every day, it would be a logistical nightmare. So, the same time every day is our policy.

I, on the other hand, was the exception as I continued to practice around my treatment, seeing patients before and after my sessions. There were a few days when trying to be a patient in between doctoring got a little more complicated than I'd anticipated, especially when consults ran longer than expected. Even though the therapists knocked on the door several times to remind me, my patient still had questions, so I continued to be a doctor, answering all their questions and concerns. By the time I emerged from the room, they had already moved on to the next scheduled patient. "We'll call you when we have the next opening. Otherwise, it'll be the end of the day," Brittany told me.

On days when I had to see patients after my treatment, it was surreal to get off the treatment table, put on my scrubs and cap, and transform back into Dr. Hwang as I walked down the hallway and into a patient room. While I was still the same doctor, something was changing inside of me as I went through radiation. When patients told me the table was hard, I knew exactly how hard. When they complained about the awkward positioning, I felt it in my own muscles. When they talked about the psychological weight of daily treatments, I understood in a way I never had before. When they reported fatigue that was not as bad as chemo but still noticeable, I knew what they meant as I laid my head down on my desk for a short catnap.

As the physical effects of radiation began to accumulate—the fatigue, the skin changes, the constant awareness of the treated area—the emotional toll surprised me the most. Each treatment was a reminder of my vulnerability, of the fundamental shift in my identity. Every time I lay on that table, I was both the doctor who understood the technology and the patient who prayed it would work.

The rhythm of treatment became a metronome for this new reality—tick, you're the doctor; tock, you're the patient. Back and forth, day after day, finding my way through this strange dance of healing and being healed.

WHEN KNOWLEDGE HURTS

Tumor board hit differently now. Sitting there, I listened to cases like I'd done hundreds of times before, but every time a patient with recurrent or metastatic cancer was presented, I would pay particular attention, noting similarities and differences between my case and theirs. In some instances, the patient clearly did not follow the recommendations, so failure was not unexpected. *You can lead a horse to water . . . ,* I'd often think. But in many other instances, the patient did everything right, followed our recommendations exactly, checked every box—and still, their cancer had returned. Under the surface, my emotions threatened to bubble up. Each case wasn't just a collection of medical data—it was a story that could be mine. Each recurrence wasn't just a statistic—it was a possibility I could no longer pretend was distant.

The medical knowledge I'd accumulated over years of practice suddenly felt less like armor and more like a burden. I knew too much. Knew about the patterns of recurrence, the survival rates, the treatment options, the cases that defied odds both good and bad.

Typically, recurrent or metastatic cases were a minority of what we saw at the breast cancer tumor board. On the day of my last treatment, however, we discussed four cases out of ten in back-to-back succession. Prior to my diagnosis, I never would have paid attention to this. I would have thought, *how unfortunate*, and then moved on to the next case. Yet on this day, the day I was finally going to finish treatment, I couldn't help but see it as an omen. *WTF? On all days to have so many of these cases?* I could have easily spiraled downward from there, but I didn't have much time because my first clinic patient was waiting.

I logged onto my computer and went through her chart. A sixty-nine-year-old female with a history of breast cancer twenty years ago. She underwent a lumpectomy followed by whole breast radiation and five years of endocrine therapy. She was doing great but started noticing neck pain. X-rays were normal, so her chiropractor did some adjustments without any improvement. An MRI of her neck showed metastatic disease in her cervical spine. In short, a twenty-year breast cancer survivor now had disease spread to her neck bones. She'd been cancer-free for two decades. Had raised her kids, celebrated anniversaries, lived her life. And now here she was, back in my office, facing a different kind of battle.

"I thought I was done with this," she said quietly. "I thought after twenty years . . ."

Her voice trailed off, but her words echoed in my head. Twenty years. Two decades of clear scans, of celebrating survivorship milestones, of gradually letting her guard down. And still, cancer had found its way back.

Before my own diagnosis, I would have processed this clinically. Would have focused on treatment options, on management strategies, on next steps. But now? Now I saw myself in her eyes. Saw my own future uncertainties reflected in her tears.

How do you counsel someone through their worst fears when they mirror your own? How do you maintain professional distance when the line between doctor and patient has become non-existent? I found myself saying the same words I'd said hundreds of times before about treatment options and new therapies. But they felt different now, weighted with personal understanding. When she asked about prognosis, about quality of life, about balancing treatment with living—I heard my own questions in hers.

The reality of my last radiation treatment hit home at that moment. It wasn't the end of breast cancer interrupting my life. I'd often tell patients to go celebrate when they finished, but those words seemed shallow now because the end of radiation meant the beginning of learning to live with uncertainty.

Once radiation ended, I would move on to the maintenance phase, taking pills for the next ten years. During this time, I would check in with my team for routine physical exams and get orders for regular scanning and blood work. But there was so much more that needed addressing. The question *What now?* kept running through my mind. It is a lens through which every future plan will be viewed. I know I can never, ever be truly free of this disease, but the real point isn't complete freedom but learning to live fully with and because of that knowledge.

RINGING THE BELL (AGAIN)

"Last day of treatment," Marie sang as she skipped into my office. "Are you ready to ring the bell?"

"I'm not ringing the bell," I said shortly. Another bell, another milestone, another moment of supposed celebration. For what?

"What's wrong?" Her tone suddenly changed. I ran her through my morning of tumor board and first clinic patient.

"That bell doesn't symbolize the last of anything. I now understand why some people don't want to ring it. Honestly, it's just the beginning . . ." My voice trailed off.

When I rang it at the end of chemo, there was no thought of the *after* crossing my mind. Being in the thick of treatment was different from being at the end of it. Now that I was at the "end," everything felt different. "No," I said quietly. "Not this time."

I could feel Marie's confusion. She'd seen me watch countless patients ring their bells and celebrate their treatment completions with genuine joy. Now here I was, refusing my own moment of triumph. This morning reminded me of how tentative these victories could be. Marie left my office, intercepting a therapist who was coming in to give me a hug. She shook her head, signaling *Now is not a good time*, and they exchanged sideways glances, clearly unsure how to handle this deviation from the script. We were all improvising now—me as a patient refusing standard ritual, them as caregivers to their own doctor.

I proceeded to my last treatment as scheduled over the lunch hour. When the beam went off, I intended to get dressed, grab lunch in the doctors' lounge, and proceed to the afternoon breast multidisciplinary clinic to counsel newly diagnosed patients. My staff, undeterred by my morning's foul mood, had other plans. Before the heavy lead door slid open, they blasted "Celebration" over the loudspeaker and danced into the room, wearing heart shaped pink glasses, and blowing noise makers. They donned me with a sash and slid sunglasses on my face. I couldn't help but smile. I loved my staff, and they loved me even when I was grumpy. They led me down the hallway to the lobby, and as the double doors swung open, all my work family and closest friends were there to celebrate the last day of radiation. Pictures were taken, the bell was rung, and together we all celebrated. I realized at that moment that I wasn't the only one on this journey. My whole staff took this journey with me, and while they weren't going through the treatment, they went through the ups and downs with me. The final day of treatment was their celebration as well.

Once all the hugs were had, I began transitioning to the next phase—monitoring, maintenance, the long road of survivorship that didn't really have an end.

As I reflected over the past few weeks, I realized that something had fundamentally changed in all of us. I'd watched my staff adapt to treating their boss and had seen them grow more comfortable with our dual relationship. I'd learned to be a patient in my own department, to accept care from people who usually took my orders. They had seen me at my most vulnerable, had helped me navigate the strange space between doctor and patient, and had taught me what it truly means to provide care.

The happiness of completing treatment was real, but so was the anxiety. Every twinge would now carry the weight of possibility. Every follow-up scan would hold the potential for life-altering news. I understood now why patients called so often with concerns I once might have dismissed as minor and felt guilt over how nonchalantly I behaved when ordering tests to evaluate those concerns.

The next day, I would return to this department as Dr. Hwang, radiation oncologist. But I would never again be just a doctor.

Every patient I saw would benefit from—or perhaps be challenged by—my deeper understanding of their journey. Definitive treatment was over, but the integration of my two identities—healer and healed—was just beginning. And this was the real milestone worth marking.

Chapter Eight
A WHOLE NEW WORLD

"I think they forgot about me," I whispered to Alicja.

We were in the waiting room of the surgery department, where we had been sitting for at least an hour. I was instructed to check in at 6:00 AM for my laparoscopic hysterectomy and bilateral salpingo-oophorectomy. At forty-six, I had two choices for managing my hormones: quarterly shots to suppress my ovaries until I officially hit menopause or surgery to remove them entirely. The math was simple—by the time I finished the shots, I'd be in natural menopause anyway. Why not just get it over with? And because the doctor was going to be in the vicinity of the uterus, I told him to take that as well so there'd be one less organ to worry about going awry on me.

"I don't want to annoy them because I'm sure they're busy, but should I go ask?" I questioned.

"This is all foreign to me. I'm always used to waiting when it comes to anything medical," Alicja reminded me. She had a good point, and not one I really thought about when being the doctor. I often don't know how long people are waiting for me, but I do tell my patients that once I'm in the room with them, they have me for as long as they need me. "Maybe call Devina," she suggested.

I dialed Devina, and she quickly answered. "What's wrong? Is everything okay?"

"Yes, everything is fine," I reassured her. "Is it normal for them to tell me to come at six and still be sitting in the waiting room at seven? Or did they forget that I'm here?"

"Oh," she laughed. "That's totally normal. We want you waiting for us, not the other way around. If they told you to be there at six, then you're the second case of the day. Once the first patient is brought back to the OR, which should be any minute because it's just past seven, they'll call you back. I'm about to scrub in for my case, but I'll be by after work."

Just as I got off the phone with her, they called my name. The next hour was kind of a blur in pre-op holding. After I changed into the hospital gown, I met the team that would be caring for me, which included the nurse, nurse anesthetist, anesthesiologist, and the gynecologic oncologist as well as his fellow. So many people . . . no wonder patients have no idea who's on their care team. After vital signs were taken, IV lines placed, saline bags hung, and pre-op questions asked, I was rolled back to the OR and told to count backward from ten as a mask was placed over my mouth and nose.

When I woke up, Alicja was sitting by the foot of my bed.

"Hey there," she said as she grabbed my toes and gave them a good squeeze. "How do you feel?"

"Excellent," I mumbled back, my mouth parched. "Let's get out of here."

"You need to pee before they will discharge you. Any chance you have to go?"

I shook my head and pointed to the nearby table that had a bottle of water on it. She opened the bottle, handed it to me, and I chugged it down. *More*, I mouthed to Alicja, who left and returned with one small can of ginger ale and one bottle of water. I drank everything and waited . . . and waited. I suddenly got the urge and went to find the bathroom, but no success. When I returned to my room, the nurse and Alicja looked at me, and I shook my head.

"Here's another can of ginger ale and water for you," the nurse said, almost anticipating that it would take more to get me to urinate. I drank them readily and tried again fifteen minutes later, with no success. When I opened the door, Alicja and the nurse were both standing there with smiles on their faces, but I shook my head again.

"One more bottle?" I asked.

I returned to the bathroom a third time, still unable to go but really wanting to be at home where I could sleep off the anesthesia in my own bed. When I got back to my room, I put a big smile on my face and said, "Let's get out of here!" For the record, I didn't technically lie, but I wasn't exactly truthful. As Alicja was driving me home, I admitted that I didn't go to the bathroom, and she just about stopped the car to return to the hospital. But I convinced her it wasn't a big deal, and they weren't going to readmit me just to have me urinate. Not trusting anything I said, Alicja called Devina and ratted me out.

"Sue!" Devina said exasperated. "Did you ever think of why they need you to go to the bathroom? What if you're in urinary retention? Then you're going to have to go back to the hospital tonight."

"Well, I figured if I had any urological issues, I would just call Steve," I quickly replied. Steve was one of my neighbors who was also a urologist.

"And what exactly do you think he's going to do for you at your house? Do you think he has a closet of catheters in his garage or something? You make no sense," she scolded me. Realizing there was nothing more I could say, I told her she was right and would be better next time, convinced there was never going to be a next time.

When we got to my house, I promised Alicja I'd call when I went to the bathroom as I shut her car door. I then crawled into my bed, where Zeus, Charlie, and Layla were happily waiting. Four hours later, I was awoken by an urge to urinate and had one of the best pees of my life. As I climbed back into bed, I thought, *Imagine being in the hospital until now, waiting to do this!*

NO REST FOR THE WEARY

"This is so stupid, but it's really addicting," I told Devina after we watched the first episode of one of her Asian teledramas. She had been watching these for a while, even paying for subscriptions to a few channels, and I laughed when she first told me. But now as I was laid up in bed, eight hours after surgery, it provided good entertainment that was totally predictable.

Devina and I were on my bed with Zeus at our feet, Layla by our heads, and Charlie in between. As she sat up to grab the remote, she noticed two small piles of vomit on the floor. "One of the dogs threw up," she sighed as she went to get paper towels and Clorox from the kitchen. "And a few more times out here," she hollered from the living room. "Based on the size of it, I think it's Charlie." That was the one good thing about having an extra-large dog, a medium dog, and a small dog. I could always tell who did it based on the size of the accident.

"Just leave it," I screamed back, too tired to deal with dog vomit. But she didn't, and after thirty minutes of deep cleaning, she rejoined me to watch another episode of the Asian drama. Halfway through, Charlie got up suddenly, making a horrible heaving noise. He then started spitting up foam and a greenish-tinged fluid all over the bedspread. Devina jumped out of bed, while I just sat there looking at my poor dog vomit for the umpteenth time. If I hadn't just had surgery, I probably would have also gotten out of bed, but I just didn't have the energy even as my bed was getting sprayed with bile and stomach acid.

"I think he needs to go to the vet. Something is wrong," Devina suggested as she stripped the comforter off the bed. I knew she was right, but sitting in an emergency vet right now was not where I wanted to be. And if I agreed, Devina would have brought him, but she had a full day of surgery tomorrow, and I didn't want her to be up all night dealing with the dog.

"He's fine, probably just ate something bad." Charlie crawled onto my lap and curled up in a ball. I stroked his head a few times, but then he sprung up again and began dry heaving.

"He is not fine, Sue. Something is really wrong." I knew she was right. I told Devina to go home and had James drive me and Charlie to urgent care. There, an X-ray of his abdomen showed a foreign body in his stomach as well as two smaller but similar appearing foreign bodies lower down in the small intestines. The vet instructed us to go to an emergency hospital because Charlie needed surgery immediately. *Of all nights to get obstructed, it has to be tonight?* I thought to myself. As tired and sore as I was, Charlie was part of the family, so James drove us to the emergency vet. We checked in at midnight and waited. Apparently, the emergency vet was not nearly as concerned as the urgent care vet. Finally, at two in the morning, I called mercy when I started developing sharp stabbing pains where my uterus used to be. It felt like my abdominal cavity was about to explode. I loved Charlie, and I tried to get him to surgery, but I wasn't even twenty-four hours out from my hysterectomy. I *really* needed to go home and lie down.

A few hours later, I called Charlie's regular vet, who wanted him brought in ASAP. James had already left for baseball training, so I drove Charlie myself even though post-op instructions recommended no driving for the next few days. I was moving slowly and had a lot of soreness in the pelvis but otherwise felt okay. I also wasn't on any pain medication other than Tylenol, so I didn't really see any absolute contraindications to driving. After dropping him off, I returned home and crawled into bed. I awoke a few hours later when the vet called with a progress report.

"I pulled out some pretty interesting stuff," she reported. "I'm actually not really sure what it is. It's some type of plastic material. Texting you a picture now to see if you can figure it out." I looked at the picture for a few seconds also unsure of what I was seeing. I could make out long thin sheets of clear and black plastic. Then it hit me. Last week, I asked James to take out four steaks from the freezer. When I got home and didn't see any steaks defrosting on the counter, I yelled at him for not doing as I asked, and he yelled back that he did. Then we looked at Zeus, who was notorious for counter surfing. As I stared at the picture from Charlie's surgery, I realized Zeus ate the meat and Charlie ate the plastic that the steaks were wrapped in. *Freaking Zeus*, I thought to myself.

"We don't have overnight services, so you need to get Charlie by six tonight. We will give him a shot of pain medication, but we recommend you take him back to the emergency vet for pain control. The first twenty-four to forty-eight hours can be rough for the pet."

I thanked her for her help but decided against returning to the emergency vet because I wasn't in the mood to sit in their waiting room for another night. When we got home, Charlie was still drowsy from the anesthesia, so I put him in my bed and fell asleep for the next few hours.

At one in the morning, Charlie woke up shrieking. "What's wrong?" I asked him as if he could respond. I tried to coax him back to sleep but he was on all fours and rigid as a board. It was clear he was in pain. *Oh my God,* I thought to myself, *I just need one restful night.* "It's okay, buddy. I know exactly how you feel," I kept repeating to him. Eventually, when the wave of pain passed, he lay down and fell back asleep. As I was about to doze off, my niece, who was on West Coast time, called. I didn't answer because I was exhausted. But she called again, at which point I picked up, concerned that something was wrong.

"Aunt Sue?" she asked.

"What's wrong?" I said half-asleep.

"They are in the kitchen fighting . . . I don't know what to do. Mom is crying a lot." My sister and her husband fought a lot from what their kids told me, but this was the first time one of them was calling me about it. The concern in my niece's voice made me worried.

"Are you guys safe?" I asked. I never would have even thought to ask this until my last visit with them earlier in the month when he got so angry that he stormed into their house screaming, "Everyone who is not my family, I want you out of this house, right now." His tone was cruel and detached. I didn't recognize it all. And even though we were all family, he was clearly referring to me, my children, and my parents. I had never seen this side of him before and didn't want to leave. But my sister, unphased, just sighed and told me to go.

"Yes, we are safe. They always just yell at each other, but mom won't stop crying this time." She fell silent as the two of us continued to listen to the fighting.

"Are you comfortable going into the kitchen?" I thought the site of their daughter would deescalate the situation.

"I can do that."

"Okay, then go into the kitchen to be there for your mom." I felt like I was telling her to go into the lion's den and didn't know if this was sound advice, but I also didn't really know what else to do short of calling the police. I started cramping again, really badly, to the point where I thought I would pass out. "Do . . . you . . . need . . . me . . . to . . . stay . . . on . . . the . . . phone . . . with . . . you?" I asked, taking deep breaths between each word. I was praying she would say no because the pain was making being on the phone unbearable.

"No, I'm good. I'm going to go out there now," she whispered. "Keep your phone on, please. I'll call you if I need you."

The intensity of the cramp eventually subsided, but I spent the rest of the night waking up to waves of pain, Charlie's high-pitched squealing, and checking my phone to see if I had any missed calls from my niece or sister.

Eventually, Charlie and I got through the night. The remainder of my recovery was uneventful, once I was able to actually rest. Charlie, on the other hand, developed an infection in the incision—while the cone was good at preventing him from licking his wound, it did nothing to stop Zeus or Layla. The poor dog had to be taken back to the operating room so the incision could be re-opened and cleaned out. But he, too, eventually recovered. My sister also recovered from that night and soon after filed for divorce.

Certainly not the way I foresaw my post-hysterectomy weekend going, but we all survived.

HELLO MENOPAUSE . . . NICE TO MEET YOU

"What do you mean I'm 165 pounds?"

I was at a routine follow-up at Sabrina's office, standing on the scale for what should have been a simple check-in. The number staring back at me didn't make sense. While I'd admittedly been more sedentary since my diagnosis, I'd also lost most of my appetite, so I was shocked to be ten pounds heavier. I strongly believed that weight maintenance was 80% diet and 20% exercise. My entire life, I followed this rule. If my clothes got a little tight, I'd eat a little less until they felt right again. My weight always normalized. Except nothing was normalizing anymore. After that day, I was more intentional about what I ate and exercised a bit more but continued to gain weight. Eventually, I turned to Amazon to order pants with elastic waistbands.

Weight is a common source of angst for breast cancer patients who are prescribed endocrine therapy. The therapy's reasoning is sound: Tumors that are stimulated by estrogen should be deprived of estrogen. But the quality-of-life implications can be unforgiving, and I never fully understood this as a premenopausal physician. When I sat across the room from follow-up patients who complained about weight gain despite their efforts to move more and eat less, I'd nod to show that I believed them even though I didn't really believe them. *Here's another woman who's not taking accountability for her actions,* I thought frequently and ended the appointment with the following recommendations: keep a food diary to accurately record intake and use an activity tracker to measure how much movement you are getting. I can only imagine how frustrated and angry these patients felt leaving the appointment because their doctor, the person they trusted to guide them on their health, didn't believe them. And now that I was the one going through it, I wondered if I wouldn't be believed.

I also wondered if this was the beginning of the end. Not to sound overly dramatic, but life is so much better without estrogen, said no woman ever. While all women will experience a significant drop in their hormones when they go through menopause, this is a gradual change that can take years. And even with the slow transition, many women struggle with the symptoms. Breast cancer, however, stripped me of the privilege of wading into the menopause pool. It was like the ten-year-old boy that impatiently waited behind my acrophobic four-year-old self, who stood at the edge of the community pool diving board looking down at the water twelve feet below. I knew it was a bad idea as I climbed up the long ladder but was too embarrassed to climb down, so I stood at the edge of the board trying to work up the courage to jump as onlookers heckled me from below. Then without warning, that ten-year-old boy pushed me from behind. As I fell into the pool below, my arms and legs flailed in all directions, and I screamed in terror. My belly and face hit the hard surface of the water with such impact that every part of my body stung like I was attacked by a thousand bees. When I climbed out of the pool, my face was bright red from being slapped by the water, my stomach burned like a grenade had exploded inside of it, and my pride was completely humiliated as children waiting in line for the diving board pointed and laughed at me. I felt like I would never recover.

And that's how I felt now. Treatment pushed me into menopause, and I didn't know how I was going to recover. Menopause. The term itself is so simple—*men* is Greek for "month" and *pausis* is Greek for "to stop". But the reality is anything but. Whether naturally or medically induced, it is a complicated experience for many women.

But it wasn't just the weight gain. It was also the hot flashes that ambushed me every thirty minutes and made my patients give me strange looks as I took off my lab coat and fanned myself with their charts while I discussed radiation complications. And the mood swings that turned me into an emotional pinball and made my kids walk on eggshells until they figured out if they were dealing with Dr. Jekyll or Mrs. Hyde. And the insomnia that made two in the morning my new laundry-folding and kitchen-cleaning time and left me yearning for a nap by noon. And the prospect of accelerated cardiovascular disease and bone loss that made me feel like I was aging overnight. And the brain fog that forced me to use my iPhone as a virtual personal assistant, reminding me of where I needed to be and when. It was the dawning realization that all women will go through this and are largely left to figure it out on their own.

The medical community's laissez-faire approach to menopause became painfully clear from the other side. When men experience low testosterone, we treat it. Slap a testosterone patch on, get those erections back, and feel like you're young again. Up until the early 2000s, hormone replacement therapy was widely offered to women to treat hot flashes that resulted from the hormonal imbalance; but in 2002, the Women's Health Initiative published data that showed it increased the risk of breast cancer, subsequently resulting in the cancellation of this treatment with no discussion of its benefits and risks. This trial has since been updated with twenty-year follow-up showing the actual risk is not nearly as high as what was previously reported; however, the medical community continues to largely steer away from hormones. As a result, when women lose their hormones, we tell them it's natural, normal, and just part of life. Deal with it. Welcome to the next phase in your life. And if you are hormone deficient from breast cancer treatment, be grateful you're cancer free and alive.

I'm not trying to make a case for hormone replacement therapy in breast cancer patients because it does increase the risk of recurrence, but I do find it interesting that aging women without breast cancer are not given the option of hormone replacement therapy given how quality of life and quality of health altering lack of estrogen can be.

Cigarettes and alcohol are known to increase the risk of breast cancer; however, women are given the option to smoke and drink if they want. Ultraprocessed foods, like chips, candy, and most fast foods are also linked to an increased risk of breast cancer, but women are given the option to buy these products every day.

The medical community has traditionally done an insufficient job of guiding women through low estrogen states because women's health is a severely neglected area of medical research and education. When I was in medical school, there was one class on menopause, and it centered around the physiologic pathology of estrogen loss in the aging female body. Aside from checking blood work and recommending calcium and vitamin D for osteoporosis and maybe vaginal estrogen for vaginal dryness, women are largely left to themselves to suck it up and "enjoy" the next phase of their life.

In the meantime, what do you do for a body that isn't following the rules anymore? The ones I'd lived by, the ones I'd prescribed to countless patients. This wasn't just about the number on the scale—it was about losing control over yet another aspect of my life. This is the one time that I was happy my phone listened to my conversations. Soon after this realization, women's health physician influencers like Dr. Marie Claire, Dr. Vonda Wright and Dr.

Jen Gunter, started popping up on my Instagram. Their message resonated with me: Women don't have to accept feeling terrible as their new normal. There are proactive measures that can be taken to reclaim your body. They provided specific recommendations on how to keep an aging female body strong and healthy. I began doing what they said and found it to be very effective. I soon passed these recommendations on to my patients who felt stuck, and they happily reported back a few months later that they finally felt unstuck.

As much joy as it brought me to hear the positive feedback from my patients, I was also embarrassed that I didn't take it upon myself to investigate these issues further before I was diagnosed. I thought about all the women who'd sat in my office over the years, complaining about symptoms I'd dismissed as minor side effects. How many times had I told them, "This is normal," when what they needed was help adjusting to the new normal. How many women had I tacitly told to just push through? The truth was I'd been part of the problem. Now I understood—this wasn't just about surviving cancer. It was about living well afterward, about maintaining quality of life, about refusing to accept diminished well-being as the price of survival. My patients deserved better. I deserved better. We all deserved better.

THE FINAL PIECE

It wasn't until months later that the full weight of what I'd done hit me. Everything that physically made me a woman—my breasts, my ovaries, my uterus—was gone. The hormones that had been part of my body's natural rhythm had been abruptly silenced. It felt unfair. The way that cancer had forced this upon me and forced me to accept a diminished quality of life as the cost of survival. I was finding a way to navigate the physical changes, but the emotional impact of these changes was much harder to process.

Well, I still have my vagina, I'd joke to myself. But everything else that made me physically female was gone. It was a strange liminal space to inhabit—still a woman but stripped down to the bare minimum needed for existence. Yet somehow, in this stripped-down version of myself, there was a new kind of strength to be found. Not in the physical markers of femininity but in the essence of what makes us women—our resilience, our ability to adapt, our capacity to find new ways of being in changed circumstances.

The surgery had taken parts of me, yes. But it hadn't taken all of me. And that was an important lesson that I learned—that womanhood isn't just about body parts or hormones. It's about who we are at our core, even when everything else has been altered or removed.

As I was coming to these realizations, everyone kept telling me how strong I was. How impressive it was that I managed work, three kids, and cancer treatment as a single parent. But the truth was I wasn't being strong—I was doing what was necessary to survive.

There's no medal for getting through cancer. No special award for continuing to parent while going through treatment. You do it because you have to, because the alternative isn't an option. What people saw as strength was just survival. But I also learned that taking care of myself wasn't selfish—it was necessary. Before, every hour spent on self-care felt like an hour stolen from my kids or my patients. A massage meant an hour not helping with homework. Playing tennis in the evening or on the weekends meant missing one of my sons' baseball games. Going on vacation meant a week of not seeing patients. The guilt was constant. Even though I worked full-time, I tried my best to be a full-time mom. And in the process, I set unrealistically high expectations for my capabilities, in turn teaching my children to have unrealistically high expectations for me as their mother.

I remember one Saturday, when heavy rain gave me an unexpected afternoon off from baseball. I was so happy because I was exhausted from the week before. All I wanted to do was watch thirty minutes of uninterrupted television, but my son, now bored because his game was cancelled for the day, wanted a ride to his friend's house. I told him to give me thirty minutes so I could relax a little, but he didn't understand why he had to wait as I wasn't "doing" anything.

"You're being lazy, Mom" he told me with disappointment. In that one instant, I felt a rage explode inside of me.

"Who are you to call me lazy? I do everything, EVERYTHING, for you and your brothers. I just want thirty minutes to myself. That is all I ask. And you have the nerve to call me lazy?" I shrieked back. I was so angry. I was so hurt. I was so unappreciated. I grabbed my car keys and drove to Alicja's house, where I spent the next hour crying hysterically because my desire to take thirty minutes for myself was perceived as laziness by my kid.

Now I understood—you can't pour from an empty cup. Taking care of myself wasn't selfish; it was essential. Not just for me but for everyone who depended on me. The hormonal changes had forced me to slow down, to listen to my body, to acknowledge its needs. In losing the physical markers of womanhood, I'd gained a deeper understanding of what it means to be whole. The real transformation wasn't the physical changes from treatment but the mental shift from seeing self-care as selfish to recognizing it as survival.

The hormone roller coaster hadn't stopped. The hot flashes still came. The weight was still there. But I was learning to ride the waves with more grace, to accept the changes while still working to improve what I could. This wasn't the journey I'd chosen, but it was the one I had, and it was making me not just a better doctor, but a better human.

THE WORRY THAT NEVER ENDS

"I need a stat MRI of my brain," I told Wassim as I got to work early one Monday morning. "Right now."

"Sue, it's the medications," he assured me. "Headaches are a common side effect." It was true that headaches were listed as a side effect for my cancer medications. But now, every twinge felt loaded with possibility.

"I've been on the meds for three months and haven't had headaches before. They started on Friday, and nothing I do is making them better. I am not a headache person, Wassim," I countered, trying to keep my voice steady.

He was in the middle of rounds, but I insisted. He stopped what he was doing and put in the order. By the end of the day, he called me when he noticed I hadn't gotten the scan.

"You made me stop my rounds to order a stat MRI. Why has it not been scheduled yet? Can they not get you in?" he asked, exasperated.

"Oh," I said sheepishly. "I got busy. And then the headache went away."

He laughed. "You're impossible."

But we both understood. This was the new normal—where every unexplained pain carried the weight of possibility, where medical knowledge was both comfort and curse. I knew the statistics, understood the probabilities, and could explain the difference between likely and unlikely symptoms. But knowing doesn't stop the fear it just gives it more detailed scenarios to work with.

Before my diagnosis, I'd tell patients to rely on mammograms and trust in early detection. Now I understood the complexity of that advice. I'd done everything as instructed and still ended up here. When they reported new headaches, breast pain, or back pain, I would gently reassure them and recommend symptomatic management for the next two weeks. If there was no improvement, then we could image. As the doctor, I knew that occasional aches and pains were normal, and imaging every patient would be overkill. As a patient, I can imagine the dread that accompanies the two-week wait. The certainties I'd once dispensed so freely had been replaced by a more nuanced understanding of this vulnerability.

When patients call about new symptoms now, I listen differently and order scans more readily because I know that reassurance doesn't cut it anymore. "It's probably just a headache" offers no comfort when you are the one with cancer.

THE TRUTH ABOUT SURVIVORSHIP

What now? This is a question I never thought about before I got diagnosed but found myself asking often once I finished radiation.

Before my cancer, when patients finished treatment, I told them, "Go ring the bell! Congratulations! You're done. Now you move onto survivorship."

When I was a resident, I did not receive any training on survivorship care and approached follow-ups from the perspective of cancer recurrence and long-term radiation complications. If patients didn't have issues with either, then they were doing great. The oncologic community, however, realized this wasn't enough as patients reported feeling abandoned by their doctors after treatment. In response, the National Cancer Institute founded the Office of Cancer Survivorship in 1996 to develop a comprehensive approach to supportive care and cancer survivorship. As a member of my institution's breast cancer leadership team, I've sat through countless meetings over the years that focused on identifying our patients' unmet needs and developing a strategy to meet these needs.

Initial efforts resulted in a survivorship binder—yes, binder. When a breast cancer patient finished treatment, she would get handed a binder that contained treatment records, office notes, doctors' contact information, a schedule of follow-up appointments, orders for imaging and labs, as well as photocopied handouts on nutrition and exercise. Aside from the fact that our handouts were photocopies of photocopies, the burden of survivorship was placed on the patient.

In early 2020, our institution founded the HEAL (**H**ealthy **E**ating and **A**ctive **L**iving) program that educated patients on the six pillars of lifestyle medicine: nutrition, physical activity, stress management, social connection, restorative sleep, and avoidance of toxic substances. It was a virtual (thanks to COVID) evidence-based support program that was a great addition to our survivorship strategy; however, the course's time commitment, limited availability, and potential out of pocket cost made its widespread roll out across the system impossible. I didn't think much more about survivorship . . . until I finished my own treatment.

While I was well versed on surveillance strategies and recommendations to reduce risk of recurrence, I completely underestimated the mental toll of treatment as well as the trauma that accompanies a cancer diagnosis. As a physician, I was always easily annoyed by early-stage patients who were overly dramatic about their diagnosis because they had an excellent prognosis. Sometimes, I wanted to say, "Please get a grip on reality, you will do fine" as they sat bawling in my office because I assumed cancer stage directly correlated with level of fear. But through my experience, I learned that stage doesn't drive fear, the ability to come to terms with *why did I get cancer* and *how do I move forward from here* does.

The trauma of being diagnosed with cancer is no different from the trauma of losing a loved one. Trauma is trauma. Life before trauma is clear and distinct, while life after trauma can be ambiguous and undefined. I found it incredibly difficult to let go of life before my diagnosis. That person—the one who didn't worry about every unexplained pain, who spent countless hours building one of the largest breast cancer programs in the city, who assumed she would always be around to see her children grow old—took a lot for granted.

But maybe letting go is not entirely bad. The person I am now understands more, feels more, connects more deeply with those around me. I'm more present in my life, more appreciative of ordinary moments, more willing to acknowledge both strength and vulnerability. It's a metamorphosis similar to that of a caterpillar becoming a butterfly. Everything is going pretty good as a caterpillar, and then one day it sheds its skin for the last time and forms a cocoon, inside of which the body will break down and form into a beautiful butterfly.

For me, everything was going well before the diagnosis, but then with the diagnosis, I had to stop life as I knew it. I was forced to slow down as I went through treatment, creating a protective bubble around me as my body was broken down to eradicate cancer. Inside my bubble, I relied heavily on close friends and family to keep me going and learned that the parts of my identity that were defined by materialism and status no longer mattered. Things that were so important to me precancer became insignificant to me once I finished treatment. As my body healed from the trauma, I emerged with a different perspective on life. Having a big house, being a top producer, and having children with straight A's were no longer my priorities. Life has a funny way of always working itself out, and I needed to clear my mind of the noise to get to a state where I could truly pursue what was important to me. My family. My friends. Myself. I no longer considered the diagnosis a curse but rather a blessing that allowed me to realize my mortality while I still have the chance to make changes and live life according to my terms, free from the judgement of others.

My practice also evolved. I still believe in evidence-based medicine and follow protocols and guidelines. But I also understand now that healing isn't just about following procedures—it's about supporting the whole person through their journey. When patients come to me now, scared about symptoms or struggling with anxiety, I don't just offer medical advice. I share what I've learned: fear doesn't mean you're weak, asking for help doesn't mean you're giving up, and living with uncertainty is possible, hard, but possible. Sometimes the best medicine isn't a scan or a prescription but the understanding that comes from someone who's walked the same path. Someone who knows that survivorship isn't just about surviving—it's about learning to live again, differently but fully.

The fear doesn't go away entirely and the awareness doesn't fade completely. But I learn to carry it differently. I allow it to inform my life without controlling it. I've developed the capacity to be both vigilant and joyful, careful and courageous, and vulnerable and secure. This is the new normal—not better or worse than the old one, just different. And for me, that's enough.

Chapter Nine

A NEW APPROACH
TO PATIENT CARE

"Why am I seeing this patient? She doesn't need radiation, Wassim." I was completely annoyed with him. My schedule was already overbooked, and he begged me to add her on.

"I need you to see her for me," he pleaded. "She's young and needs chemo, but she's refusing." He paused for a few seconds. "She's scared, Sue. I need you to show her that you survived and so can she."

I was still annoyed since I didn't see how my personal experience was going to change this patient's mind. As a team, we occasionally saw patients who cherry-picked their treatment despite what was recommended, and it frustrated us because the more they deviated from the standard of care, the more they put themselves at risk of recurrence. Most agreed to surgery, some refused chemo, some refused radiation, some refused endocrine therapy, and on rare occasions some refused all of it. As oncologists, we offered guidance and made recommendations, but the patient had to decide what they were willing or capable of enduring. If I couldn't convince a patient to follow the treatment plan with my expertise as a doctor, I wasn't quite sure how my patient experience would convince them.

I reviewed her chart and learned that she was forty-two years old with two children, ages twelve and eight, who was found to have breast cancer on her routine mammogram. She decided to undergo a mastectomy, but chemotherapy was recommended before surgery because of the size and biology of the tumor. As I entered her room, I felt like a fish out of water because she wasn't there to hear my standard radiation script, and for the first time since being a resident, I struggled to find the words to start the conversation.

"Well, this sucks," I said matter-of-factly. It was something I thought often when I met young patients but never actually said . . . until now.

She laughed in response. She was clearly still in shock from her earlier appointment with Wassim. Her eyes were swollen and puffy from crying. Redness still lingered, but there were no tears. She was emotionally drained, having cried all her tears when she found out she needed chemo.

"I'm not quite sure how to start this visit," I admitted. "I know Dr. Mchayleh is really thorough, so I don't want to talk about that stuff if you don't want me to." She nodded in agreement.

"Do you have any questions for me?" She shook her head. With no guidance about how to approach this consultation, I figured I would continue to ask yes or no questions until she was ready to say more.

"Have you told your family yet?" She shook her head no.

"It will be hard to break this news, but I can offer some tips on how to do it, when you're ready. Do you have kids?" She nodded and held up two fingers.

"Are they young?" She nodded. I knew the answer but was hoping talking about kids would break the ice.

"Kids are amazingly resilient and can be surprisingly helpful," I joked. No response—she was staring at the floor. "I know as moms we try to protect them from the world but sometimes letting them see bits and pieces of the real world is good for them."

There was no acknowledgement of what I'd said. I wasn't sure if she was even listening. I knew she was going through a lot, but I was starting to feel uncomfortable. It reminded me of going on an awful first date where I had to keep asking the guy questions to avoid the awkward silence. But unlike the date, I couldn't get a fake telephone call and leave. I changed my approach and decided to sit in silence with her until she was ready to speak because the twenty-questions approach was getting me nowhere.

"I don't want treatment," she finally said after what felt like an eternity.

"What worries you about chemo the most?"

"All of it." She started to get choked up.

"I get it. No one ever wants chemo. But can you tell me what you are most worried about?" I've found through the years that many patients will say no, but the reasons varied greatly. Sometimes they don't know how they're going to pay for it. Sometimes they can't afford to be sick because they're the primary caregiver for their children and/or elderly parents. Sometimes they're afraid they'll lose their job if they take time off from work. Sometimes they don't want to lose their hair. At this point in my career, I assumed nothing.

"He says I'll get through it and that complications are rare, but how does he know? If a complication is going to happen, it's going to happen to me," she scoffed.

I thought of my precancer response, which was to use probabilities and statistics to reassure. But my patient experience taught me how poorly numbers can reassure anyone, no matter how favorable they are. I remembered vividly foreseeing that I would develop every major complication. The fear was palpable and completely paralyzing. The emotional side of my brain completely overtook the rational side, and all the knowledge I'd accumulated from my years of practicing medicine fell to the wayside. But after getting over the shock, my rational side was able to kick back in. I just had to figure out a way to tap into hers.

"Did Dr. Mchayleh tell you why he was sending you to me?" She nodded her head in response. "When he recommended chemo to me, I was in such denial. I got second opinions even though I knew he was right. I also thought I was going to get every complication, and there was nothing he could say to me to make me feel better."

I was about to tell her I got through it and so would she . . . but I paused.

"Even though I'm a breast cancer doctor, I was terrified of treatment. And it was hard for me to understand the fear that my patients had from the sidelines. So right now, I'm talking to you as a patient, and I'd like to share my chemo experience with you if you would find that helpful."

Over the next thirty minutes, I informed her about how helpful steroids can be for midnight laundry folding sessions, recommended some Netflix shows to watch when too tired to get out of bed, told her how self-sufficient kids can become when they know Mom isn't feeling well, and recounted other unexpected but funny realizations during treatment. It was nice to hear her laugh, and after a while, she opened up and talked about all her fears. As she talked, I just sat there and listened. I didn't try to reassure her. I didn't try to sweep her fears to the side. I just sat there and acknowledged what she was saying. At the end of the appointment, she thanked me for my time and asked me if she could give me a hug.

"Of course," I replied as I held out my arms.

"I'm sorry you had to go through this," she said softly as we embraced. "But I want you to know that your opinion matters so much more to me because you have been where I am going. You've seen it from both sides. You get it, and I know that you get me."

As I walked back to my office, I kept thinking about what she said. *You have been where I am going.* My diagnosis gave me a deeper understanding of the complexities of both the disease and the patients with the disease. They often describe breast cancer as a sisterhood—a club that no one ever wants to join. Up until this point, I considered my greatest value to be my knowledge as a breast cancer doctor, but this patient showed me that my personal experience can be just as, and in some cases more, important.

Just then I got a text from Wassim. "She agreed to chemo. THANK YOU   "

From that point on, I found myself navigating a strange new reality. Patients would come in for their radiation consultations, often newly diagnosed, scared, and looking for answers. I'd sit across from them, trying to find the right balance between empathy and expertise.

"What's it really like?" one patient asked me directly, having followed me on Instagram. "Not the medical stuff—the real stuff."

I paused, considering. A month ago, I would have given my standard answer about side effects and success rates. Now? Now I knew about struggling with drain management and all the possible options to deal with chemo-induced hair loss. But I also knew about the Boobie Fairy showing up at your door, about friends organizing meal trains and other supportive services, about discovering strength you didn't know you had.

Initially when I started seeing patients after sharing my diagnosis on social media, I made an intentional effort to keep my patient counseling on the professional side, informing them of procedural details, complications, and outcomes. I felt that if I opened up too much as a patient, the doctor/patient relationship would be compromised. But I found that my patients were more interested in my patient opinion because that was the side that made me relatable and made them trust me more as their doctor. That was the side that opened them up to undergoing treatments that they truly did not want to do, and that was the side that understood all their concerns on the most visceral level.

"I just want to feel normal again," my next patient, Mrs. B, said, eyes welling with tears.

She was a lively seventy-year-old patient who'd completed radiation three years prior, and I knew her well, seeing her every six months since the end of her treatment. This visit felt different, though. Three months after completing my own treatment, I had a different level of empathy for her as I listened to her continue to struggle with the all-too-common symptoms of endocrine therapy—weight gain, mood swings, and fatigue. I pulled out my prescription pad and started writing instructions for her. I tore off the paper and handed it to her for review.

"I am prescribing strength training twice a week. You can go to the gym, or you can buy a set of dumbbells for your home— nothing too heavy, start with ten pounds at most. While you are watching TV, get into a routine of working with the dumbbells for thirty minutes, twice a week."

Mrs. B's demeanor changed as I gave her instructions. She was listening intently, trying to absorb every word I said.

"I also want you to walk three times a week for thirty minutes at a brisk pace. You don't need to do crazy cardio. Just get outside and walk. Now this next item—" I pointed at the prescription I handed her. "Do you know how much protein you eat a day?"

"Well, it's typically Greek yogurt for breakfast, some type of meat on top of my salad for lunch, and then a piece of fish or chicken for dinner," she replied.

"That's not enough. If I had to guesstimate, it sounds like you are eating about sixty grams at best, and you really should be at 130 grams a day based on your height. It's important to know your macros and make sure you are taking in enough protein. We are shooting for one gram per pound of ideal body weight because you don't have enough muscle on your frame. Your body has no estrogen now, and if you don't get enough protein, your muscles will waste away. It's a condition called sarcopenia, and it's very common in older women. What we need to do now is steer your ship in a different direction, and with a little bit of education, we can reverse this. I know protein is the buzzword now, but it's critical for you. You won't be able to maintain muscle if you don't have the basic building blocks of muscle. Got it?" She nodded in understanding.

"Okay, now onto fiber. Make sure you are getting a lot of fresh fruits and vegetables in your diet. You want about twenty-five grams of fiber—not only does it keep you regular, but it helps to stabilize your blood sugar and can possibly reduce hot flashes. Fiber is your friend. This last thing I wrote, creatine. Do you know what that is?" She shook her head.

"Creatine is an amino acid that helps with muscle building and keeps our bones strong. But it may also help with fatigue and the brain fog that happens with endocrine therapy. The target is five grams a day. Ideally, you want to try to eat your nutrition, but if you can't, it's okay to supplement."

"This is so helpful. Thank you so much . . ." She hesitated before completing her sentence. "I don't want to offend you, but can I ask you a question?"

I nodded.

"Why didn't you tell me this before?"

"I didn't know this before. Actually, I didn't bother to learn this before," I admitted. "I considered side effects to be an acceptable trade off to being cancer free and didn't think it was a big deal because everyone talks about how miserable menopause is. And then after I got diagnosed and experienced the misery firsthand, I started looking for other options."

"I'm embarrassed to say that it took me getting breast cancer to learn more about how to manage symptoms related to endocrine therapy. It's been a very interesting journey, to say the least. There's so much information out there about how to better manage these symptoms, but you have to know where to look. My diagnosis has taught me that it doesn't have to be this way. And now, I just want my patients to know that it doesn't have to be this way."

Mrs. B was shocked by my candidness. She took my hands in hers and squeezed them tightly as her eyes welled up with tears.

"I finally feel heard. You are right. It doesn't have to be this way. Thank you so much."

NO ONE IS PROTECTED

"Can you just see her to see her?" Devina asked me over the phone. "This is her third recurrence. She'll let me excise the tumor but continues to refuse anything more. She won't do a mastectomy, she won't do radiation, and she doesn't want endocrine therapy. But I need you to just see her so we can document that you've had the discussion."

Devina was clearly frustrated, and I understood why. One day, this patient won't have a recurrence in her breast. Instead, she'll have it in her body, and when that happens, she'll die of breast cancer.

"Send her over now. I'll add her on."

When I met the patient in my clinic, she was accompanied by her daughter and husband, who both looked completely frustrated with her. I went through my standard spiel about the necessity of radiation after a lumpectomy or a completion mastectomy to give her the best possible shot at local control.

"I know what the recommendations are. But I'll continue to roll the dice. I don't want radiation, and I don't want to lose my breast," she said confidently.

"You are aware that this cancer can spread to other parts of your body?" I questioned.

"It hasn't yet," she replied.

"Yet," I interjected. "You are gambling with your life. Early-stage breast cancer is treatable and curable. One day it won't be curable."

"You sound like you are reading from Dr. McCray's script," she said sarcastically.

"That's because we've seen patients die of breast cancer, and it's a horrible way to go. You clearly care about this cancer to some degree since you're willing to have mammograms and you're willing to let Dr. McCray take out the tumor. So what is stopping you from taking the next step?"

She didn't have a snarky reply. She sat there quietly with no response.

"She's scared," her daughter spoke up. "She's scared of treatment."

"I understand your fear," I told her, touching my head where a wig covered my regrowth. "I just finished treatment for breast cancer. I got it all, mastectomies, chemo, and radiation."

She laughed at the irony, "A breast cancer doctor that gets breast cancer? I guess no one is protected from this disease." She gave me a look over and then questioned, "Are you joking? You don't look like a cancer patient."

"This is a hair topper." I lifted the topper to show her my bald head. "I lost most of my hair from chemo, despite doing my best to try to save it. And these"—I pointed to my chest—"These are implants."

I could tell the irony of my situation hit her and sensed a change in her demeanor.

"You are right. No one is guaranteed anything when it comes to cancer. Despite spending everyday counseling patients through treatment, I was terrified. And even though I'm on the other side of it now, I still get scared at times. You've been so lucky that this cancer keeps coming back in the breast. But if you ever are unfortunate enough to develop metastatic disease, you will regret not doing everything in your power when you had the chance to because as scary as treatment is, dying of metastatic breast cancer is by far scarier." I paused and let what I said sink in.

For the first time that day, she really looked at me. The questions poured out—not just about procedures and side effects, but about fear, about pain, and about daily life during treatment. After an hour of real conversation, she agreed to surgery.

"Schedule her for a completion mastectomy before she changes her mind," I texted Devina.

"Strong work   ," she replied.

SURVIVORSHIP GOES BEYOND SURVIVAL

The transformation in my practice wasn't just about being more empathetic—though that was part of it. It was about refusing to accept diminished quality of life as the inevitable cost of survival and recognizing that "You're lucky to be alive" isn't an adequate response to legitimate struggles with treatment side effects.

For too long, the medical community approached treated patients with a focus on monitoring for recurrence while considering side effects minor inconveniences. But that's not the way forward. I realized these "inconveniences" shaped every aspect of survivors' daily lives. They deserved more than sympathy. They deserved solutions. My own experience taught me that survival wasn't enough. We all deserved a chance to live well and thrive.

To make it happen, I started surveying my patients about what worked for them, collecting their wisdom and experiences. Every appointment became an opportunity to learn as well as teach.

"Now that I've finished treatment," I'd say, "I find myself wondering what's next. How did you handle this part?"

Their answers surprised me. Women who were years ahead of me in their survivorship journey had developed strategies I'd never considered, found solutions that no medical textbook wrote about. One patient showed me breathing techniques that helped with anxiety. Another shared her method for managing hot flashes with acupuncture.

By asking these questions and acknowledging that I too was on this journey, I discovered something powerful: When patients feel heard, they are more likely to speak up, share their struggles, and actively engage in their recovery. And the results were tangible. Women who'd been fighting weight gain for years started seeing changes. Those battling fatigue found new energy. The vague promises of "It gets better with time" were replaced with action-able steps and measurable progress.

I learned to treat the whole person, not just the disease and to acknowledge that recovery is about regaining a life worth living, just as much as it is about clear scans and good blood work. The path forward required recognition that a great life is possible after cancer and implementation of changes to move the needle forward. The changes weren't revolutionary—most of the information had been available all along. This was a different kind of medicine than what I'd practiced before. The medical knowledge I'd accumulated over years of practice was still crucial, but now it was informed by personal experience, enriched by patient wisdom, and shaped by a deeper understanding of the recovery process.

"Everyone tells me I need to stay positive," a patient shared during a follow-up visit. "But sometimes I just want to say, 'This really sucks,' and I want someone to acknowledge that this is hard."

I thought about all the times I'd encouraged patients to "stay positive" before my own diagnosis. Now I understood—positivity wasn't about denying fear or difficulty. It was about finding ways to live alongside them.

"It is hard," I agreed. "And it's okay to say that."

The relief on her face was immediate. Sometimes the greatest gift we can give each other is permission to be honest about our struggles. Not to wallow in them but to acknowledge them, process them, and then figure out how to move forward.

The medical profession is slowly changing, moving toward more comprehensive care models. But change takes time, espe-cially when every modification must be evidence-based, proven, verified, and then adopted by practitioners. This pace at which the medical community adopts change makes the sloths working at the DMV in *Zootopia* appear lightning fast. Case-in-point: the

National Cancer Institute initially introduced the idea of survivorship in the late 1990s. This concept has finally become commonplace at large academic and medical institutions, who have the resources to deploy for multidisciplinary survivorship care. But the smaller, community-based clinics are still behind.

Sometimes the fastest way to improve outcomes is to identify the deficiencies from personal and patient experiences and seek out the evidence to improve outcomes, even if that evidence is not yet commonplace or widely known. My practice had become a laboratory for these changes. Each success story, each improvement in quality of life, added to the growing evidence that we could do better—that we needed to do better—in supporting cancer survivors for all types of cancer.

At the end of the day, medicine isn't just about extending life, it's about making that life worth living. And this is the most important lesson cancer taught me as both doctor and patient: Survival is just the beginning. Real healing comes in learning to live fully again.

Chapter Ten

LESSONS ON FEAR, FAITH, AND MOVING FORWARD

The sunset painted the baseball field in shades of orange and gold. From my usual spot by right field, I could hear the distinctive ping of the bats, the umpire's calls echoing across the diamond, and my son's high school team cheering from the dugout. Normally, I'd be answering emails or checking patient charts—multitasking through another evening of baseball. But something about the sunset over the outfield made me pause and really look at the scene before me. *How many games had I sat through without really seeing them? How many moments had I missed while focusing on the next obligation?*

For the first time in years, I wasn't thinking about what needed to be done next. I was just . . . here. Present. Watching my son play the game he loved under a sky that seemed determined to remind me how beautiful ordinary moments could be.

A strange sense of calm settled over me. Not because everything was perfect—it wasn't. Not because I wasn't afraid anymore—I was. Hell, I *am*. But because I finally understood that the beauty in the ordinary and the ability to stay in the present are what surviving is all about.

THE STRENGTH IN SHOWING UP

"Mom, I'm ready to go," Sam announced, surprising me one Monday morning. After a grueling weekend tournament where his team played five games in two days in scorching temperatures, I expected him to skip baseball academy the following day because his body was understandably sore.

"Are you sure?" I asked in disbelief. "I don't want you to overdo it."

"Yeah, but I'm not going to get any better if I don't keep pushing through," he said matter-of-factly. "I'm not in pain, it's just soreness," he reassured me.

I was speechless. This was my middle son, the one who needed constant reminders about homework and required three wakeup calls before coming out of his room. And now he was standing before me ready to go. *Where did this come from?* I thought to myself.

For years, I've told him that most of the battle was just showing up and got so frustrated and angry when he couldn't work up the energy to just show up. Now he was showing me that that he understood—not just being present physically but being committed to growth even when it was uncomfortable and easier to stay home.

My kids had a front row seat to my health drama, watching me navigate cancer treatment while maintaining my practice and pushing through fatigue to keep our family's rhythm. But rather than cover their eyes in fear, they recognized what was happening and learned from it. They saw what resilience looked like firsthand and were now emulating it.

Recently, James traveled with his high school baseball team to Las Vegas for a tournament. While many parents accompanied the team, I stayed behind but was able to watch the games on the Perfect Game TV livestream. When James got up to bat, the announcer said my name, which caught me off guard. I turned up the volume to hear, "James shares that his mom inspires him to be strong and persevere." I was surprised and touched by this because James is a very stoic individual. Since he started driving, I saw him less and less as he would leave for school at 6:45 AM and sometimes not return home until 10 PM. Afraid that we would drift apart, I started kissing him on the cheek and telling him that I loved him before he left for school in the morning. He would respond with an "okay" and shut the door on his way out. There was no reciprocating hug, or I love you, just an okay. But I guess even cancer has a way of breaking down walls and teaching children lessons, no matter how old and independent they appear to be.

After my diagnosis, I did interviews with several local news stations to share my story and promote breast cancer awareness in the community. One of the reporters, who was also a breast cancer survivor, commented that I was a superwoman and asked me where I got my strength. I took a few seconds to answer because I never would have used the word strong to describe myself during this time. I told her I was just trying to get by. The world didn't stop when I got cancer. Even though I slowed down, everything else kept going full steam ahead. My dogs still expected breakfast at six, my kids still had to leave for school at seven, and my clinic still started promptly at eight. So how did I survive? I showed up. I may have felt like crap, but I was still there. I learned firsthand that strength isn't just defined by invincibility; it's also defined by showing up, day after day, and doing what needs to be done.

Sometimes the greatest lessons we teach aren't the ones we plan but the ones we live.

It's also true that life has a way of teaching us what we need to learn whether we want the lesson or not. Cancer taught me that being present isn't just about physically showing up; it's about truly experiencing the moments you're in. Like that evening at the baseball field, when the sunset caught my attention and held it. Now I understood—tomorrow isn't guaranteed for anyone. But there will always be this moment. Now, when Nathan comes to watch TV in my room, I actually watch with him instead of working on my laptop. When James wants to talk about baseball, I listen—*really* listen—instead of just nodding along.

These aren't particularly earth-shattering changes. They aren't even super visible ones. But they have been profound in their own way because they've taught me that the beauty of life happens in these in-betweens—the ordinary conversations, the routine activities, the daily rituals we all take for granted. Cancer had taken things from me, yes. But it has given me the understanding to appreciate the small things.

I spent a lot of time during my treatment yearning for my life precancer, wishing at night to return to the person I once was, willing to trade almost anything for that chance. But I have since come to terms with the fact that life after cancer isn't about returning to who you were because that person is gone. It's about becoming someone new, someone who understands both fragility and strength in deeper ways. The physical changes are permanent: the scars, the hormone changes, the constant awareness of my body's vulnerabilities. But the emotional and spiritual changes have been more profound: the wisdom to know what truly matters, the courage to live fully even with uncertainty. Cancer has been a blessing for me, a blessing that teaches me fully about my mortality, while I am still able to make changes for a better, more fulfilling future.

FOR LOVE OF THE GAME

I've always had a love-hate relationship with tennis. I was introduced to the sport as a young child, played four years on my high school team, and then recruited to Wellesley College where I played another four years at the D3 collegiate level. But then life got in the way. First it was medical school and residency in downtown Chicago, where a tennis court was hard to come by and free time was even harder to find. Then it was my kids and an attending radiation oncology job that left me with no downtime. Even though I didn't play, I thought about it and missed it . . . a lot. As my kids grew older and more independent, I was able to dip my toes back in. While muscle memory preserved my strokes, the twenty-year hiatus was unforgiving on my mental game and physical stamina. It was so frustrating that I would start, then stop, then start, then stop again.

I loved playing, I loved winning even more, but I hated losing the most. This mentality affected my confidence to play with people I didn't know and prevented me from joining local tennis teams, which I knew I needed to do to improve my competitiveness. I confined myself to hitting with instructors and Dave, who had the most carefree personality and didn't care how I hit so long as I was willing to join him for a drink afterward. Eventually, Dave convinced me to play with some of his friends, but I still limited my playing circle because of how much I hated to lose.

And then cancer came along and reframed everything. I went from worrying about losing to worrying about whether I'd ever be able to play again. I didn't know if complications from surgery or radiation would cause the muscles of my chest wall and shoulder to scar down and limit my range of motion and ability to hit the ball. As I grappled with the possibility of never playing again, I was suddenly okay with losing because losing meant that I was playing.

Once I recovered from surgery, I joined three teams and got back on the court every chance I got. I lost . . . a lot. But I was so thankful for each and every one of those losses. Every defeat was an opportunity to learn and improve. Each serve, each rally, each match became something to appreciate rather than just accomplish. I was reminded to focus on the process and not the outcome.

For my first 8.0 level mixed doubles match, I was paired with a partner who had just recovered from rotator cuff surgery. Because neither of us were in top form, I assumed this match was going to go in the L column. Amazingly though, we both managed to rally and refused to give up. It ended up being a marathon—two and a half hours against a pair who'd played together for five years and never lost. We won . . . but barely. Despite being completely beat up, I was proud of myself for working within my limitations and figuring out how to succeed.

I was feeling so happy until I woke up the next morning and couldn't lift my shoulder. The rational doctor in me knew exactly what this was—I played an intense match, left everything on the court. Of course I was sore. This was normal postexercise pain.

But cancer changes how you interpret "normal."

Three days passed, and the pain persisted. My doctor brain kept saying, *Muscle strain, ordinary inflammation, expected recovery.* My patient brain whispered, *What if it's not? What if the tennis just made me notice something that was already there?*

A week of internal debate followed. *Should I tell Wassim? Should I get an MRI?* I tried to be rational, but rationality doesn't always win against fear.

Finally, on day seven, the pain disappeared as suddenly as it had come. Just muscular soreness after all. But that week of worry had taught me something about living in this new reality—where the guard never fully comes down.

The shoulder pain was a turning point. After that week of worry, I had to confront an uncomfortable truth: I couldn't live the rest of my life suspecting cancer in every ache. I needed to find a balance between vigilance and paranoia. It helped that I saw success stories every day in my practice—women living full lives five, ten, twenty years out from diagnosis. Yes, sometimes cancer came back, like my patient whose cancer had returned in her bones after twenty years. But more often, it didn't.

The statistics I'd quoted to patients for years took on new meaning. That eighty-five percent ten-year survival rate wasn't just a number anymore—it was a community I belonged to, a group of women learning to live with uncertainty while refusing to be defined by it. I started playing more tennis, not less. Started making plans further into the future. Not because I was certain everything would be fine, but because I understood now that certainty was never guaranteed—for anyone, cancer survivor or not.

I was learning to live fully even when life feels fragile. Because that's what surviving really means: not just making it through treatment but learning to live again on the other side.

GRIEVING WITH GRACE

"Can you please meet me at Gery's house now?" I half-asked, half-commanded Devina.

"Yes," she replied, understanding the urgency of the situation when she heard my frantic tone.

I had just gotten a text from my ex-husband's friend that read, "I don't know if I'm overreacting here, but the guard house just called me because Gery hasn't answered their calls all day and there is a vendor that has been trying to get into the neighborhood." I wasn't particularly concerned until Sam told me that he hadn't heard from his father in two days. Sam was incredibly close to Gery, exchanging a text or a brief hello almost every day. This prompted me to grab my phone and dial his number; his phone rang and rang with no answer. I then asked the boys to call him and still no answer. I developed an unsettling feeling, grabbed my car keys and headed to his home.

I knew Gery hadn't been feeling well and had been in and out of the hospital for the past six months, getting every conceivable test known to mankind. When I asked what was going on, he said they were still trying to figure it out. I didn't pry because while we communicated well when it came to the kids, we didn't have a close relationship. He was always the fun parent, and I was the reliable one. Even though the parenting plan established at the time of our divorce stipulated that the boys divide their days equally between both parents, they gravitated towards my home most of the time and he never made them feel bad about that. I, on the other hand, grew resentful over the years, as carrying most of the parental responsibilities left me exhausted and overwhelmed. Consequently, I chose to never engage in conversation with him if it wasn't about the boys.

As I pulled up to his house, Devina was already waiting in the driveway. I rang the doorbell. No answer. I knocked hard on the door. No answer. I then entered the keypad code to unlock the front door.

"Gery?" I called out. "Are you here? I tried calling but you didn't answer. Devina and I are coming in," I announced as we stepped into the foyer of his home. I continued to walk further in as Devina remained planted in the foyer with a look of worry and fear clearly written all over her face. Seeing that she did not want to go any further, I wandered through the house alone. His home was how it always was, clean and tidy with nothing out of place. His bedroom door was closed, so I knocked loudly and called out his name again. No response.

"Gery, I'm coming in," I said firmly as I opened his door. His bed was unmade, which was unusual for him. I walked through the bedroom into the master bathroom and then through the remainder of his house. There was no sign of him. I then peaked my head into his garage, only to be disappointed when I saw his parked car.

"He's not here," I reported back to Devina, who had left the house and was sitting on the driveway. I sat down beside her and decided it was time to call the police for help. As I filed a missing person report, Devina stood up, looking intently at the house.

"Call his phone, Sue," she said softly. I gave her a questioning look as I picked up my phone to dial him again. *Ring, ring, ring, ring.* The phone was ringing from inside the house. I re-entered the home and followed the sound to his master bedroom, where his phone was ringing from the nightstand. I then walked around the foot of the bed and found his lifeless body in the small space between the other side of the bed and the bedroom wall.

I ran out of the house screaming to Devina. The next few hours were a blur. The paramedics and police arrived. Once he was declared dead, the paramedics drove off and more police arrived. Devina and I sat shocked on his driveway.

"We need tell the boys," Devina said gently. "I'll asked Q to come here so we can figure out how to tell the boys." Soon Q pulled up to the curb. He got out of his car and gave me a big hug. For the first time since I met him, he had no words. I could barely process what was happening myself. While I served as the primary caregiver, Gery was always there if the boys needed something. When I got diagnosed, I thought to myself *at least the boys still have their father if something happens to* me. Now my safety net was gone, and I was the only parent they had left. How was I going to tell my boys that their father is dead? They were just finding their bearings again after watching me go through cancer treatment. How could life be this cruel? What did they do to deserve this?

As we drove to my home, I kept running through opening lines in my head; it eerily reminded me of that day James and I were driving, and I was trying to figure out how to tell him I had cancer. When we got to the house, I called all the boys into the living room. Knowing that I had gone off to look for their father, they knew something was wrong the moment they saw Devina and Q.

"Your father is gone," I heard myself say.

Sam sat down on the couch and put his head in his hands. James stood by Q, arms folded, staring blankly at me. Nathan looked at me, then Devina, then Q, almost as if he was waiting for the punchline to a really bad joke. Soon, James started asking questions. "What happened? Where was he found? Why didn't he call for help? How long was he there?" I tried to answer him the best I could, but Q thankfully took over because I wasn't making much sense. Sam had quiet tears and regret. "I should have spent more time with him." Devina moved next to him on the couch and rubbed his back.

Nathan headed to his room. I got up to follow, but he shut the door on me before I could enter. He let out a guttural scream followed by sounds of deep sobbing. I leaned my back against the outside of his door, slid down to the floor, and covered my ears with my hands, trying to buffer the sound of my child in horrific pain. I wanted to go in, hug him and tell him that it would be okay, but I knew I also had to let him get these emotions out. As a mother, I have never experienced anything more painful than hearing my child sob from the other side of a closed door and be able to do nothing.

The next morning the boys were up early and asked to go to his house. While they were clearly still in shock, I thought taking them over there would help them come to terms with their new reality. When they entered his home, they immediately headed in separate directions. Sam went to his walk-in closet and closed the door. James quietly sat down in front of his computer and went through old photos. Nathan walked through the rooms looking at all the sports memorabilia that they had spent years collecting. After an hour, they emerged with items they wanted keep, loaded them in the trunk of my car, and drove back in silence.

When we reached my house, they unloaded the car and sequestered themselves in their rooms for the remainder of the day. I didn't really know what to do with myself. In many ways, trying to come to terms with his death reminded me of trying to come to terms with my breast cancer diagnosis. While everything still looked the same around me, nothing felt the same anymore. I knew the world would keep on going with patients needing to be seen and homework needing to be done, while our lives were placed on temporary pause so that we could recover from his death.

Andrea called me later in the day to check in. "They haven't really come out of their rooms," I informed her. "I knock every few hours to check in, but they aren't talking much. I want to give them space."

"I think you are doing the right thing," she agreed. "I just wanted to tell you how impressed I am with James through all of this."

"What do you mean? What did he do?" I asked, having no idea what she was talking about.

"Alden texted him to see if he needed anything and James said he was doing okay and would get through this. But he asked Alden to be kind to Sam and Nathan because they were struggling and really missed their father." I started to tear up as I heard this. Even though he was grieving too, James was more concerned about his brothers and getting them through this. For years, James had a bad case of oldest child syndrome; no matter how hard I would plead with him to be kinder to his brothers, he would always sarcastically inform me, "I was fine as an only child mom. I didn't ask you to have more children." But with the sudden passing of his father, he seemed to have matured overnight, prioritizing his brothers' well-being over his.

The first full day after his death drew to a close and I started turning off all the lights in the house. Sam and Nathan suddenly emerged from their rooms asking for a ride to the Marucci Clubhouse, a twenty-four-hour baseball training facility. I was surprised by their request but gladly obliged because I wanted to get them out of the house. When we pulled up to the facility at 10 PM, we were the only car in the parking lot.

"Give us an hour, okay mom?" Sam said before he shut the door. I sat in the car, in the dark, in total silence. Time flew by because before I knew it, Nathan was climbing back into the car.

"How was it?" I asked him. He shrugged his shoulders as he took a swig of water.

"Sam needs a few more minutes," he reported to me. He then paused for a bit before speaking. "His eyes were red. I think he was crying as he was hitting so I left to give him some time to himself. Do you think it's okay to leave him alone?"

I nodded, unable to speak as tears started streaming down my cheeks. I heard Nathan texting on his phone. Once he sent the message, he said, "I just told Dad that Sam really misses him. I told him that I really miss him too and that we finished batting at Marucci. I think it would make him happy to know that we're playing baseball right now. Do you think it's okay if I keep texting him? I think he can read them from Heaven."

I remained silent, doing my best to slow down the tears. I was so sad for my children, but also so impressed by Nathan's emotional maturity. He knew that Sam needed space and gave it to him. He knew that his dad was still around, even though his body was gone. When did my twelve-year-old get so wise?

"It's okay to cry mom," he whispered in my ear as he hugged me from behind.

The next day was spent the same way. Boys in their room during the day, followed by a late-night visit to Marucci Clubhouse.

As we headed into the weekend, I expected them to lay low. Sam was registered for a Perfect Game Baseball Showcase, one that he had been looking forward to for months because it was qualifier for the "Naties" (a.k.a. Nationals). But I thought for sure he would skip it because he wasn't in any emotional condition to perform. When he woke me up at 6 AM that Saturday morning dressed and ready to go, I was shocked. My child, who had every reason in the world to not show up, decided to show up. And three days after receiving the most devastating news of his life, he was still able to perform at the top of his game, being named a 2025 Perfect Game Sunshine East Prospect Gateway Top Prospect and earning an invite to Nationals.

The weekend ended with the wake. We arrived at the funeral home a few minutes early so the boys could say their goodbyes before everyone arrived. The scent of fresh flowers drifted throughout the funeral home, reminding me of my living room in the days that immediately followed the mastectomies. We were about to walk into the viewing room when Nathan stopped just outside the doorway, biting on the neckline of his polo. He wanted to see his father one more time, but I could tell he wasn't quite ready to face the reality that was waiting for him in the room.

Margaret, who dropped everything and flew in to support me as soon as she heard the news, and Devina stayed with him as I entered the room with James and Sam. We approached his body together and I held their hands tightly in mine as if they were little boys trying to cross a busy street. James and Sam stood frozen by the open casket, their eyes locked on their father's still face, struggling to accept that they would never hear his voice again. Sam swallowed hard, trying to be strong but feeling utterly lost, while James studied every line on his face, knowing this would be the last time he would ever see him. As I put my hands on their backs, I turned my head to see Nathan peaking his head in. I could see he was working up the courage to see his father one last time.

The funeral home soon filled with family, friends, teachers, coworkers, and baseball teammates. Through the quiet hum of voices, occasional laughter would break through as people recounted funny memories. The village that once supported my family through my breast cancer diagnosis returned to support us once again. Even though the boys were deep in their grief, their village reminded them that they were so loved and would never be alone. Their presence became a guiding light for my children, helping to lift the weight of their loss and bring comfort in times of despair.

I know it will take my children years to fully process the death of their father, but I have been amazed so far by how they have handled themselves. As they stood witness to my breast cancer journey, they developed a set of coping skills that helped them navigate the sudden passing of their father. By continuing to show up for them through the exhaustion, pain and uncertainty of treatment, I taught them how to face hardship with courage. These lessons carried them forward, allowing them to grieve with grace for their father. They leaned on each other and looked out for each other, becoming closer in the process and honoring his memory with love and determination.

A Fresh Perspective, With Staying Power

"Do you ever stop being scared?" a newly diagnosed patient asked me.

"No," I answered honestly. "I still panic with every little pain. But I'm doing a better job learning to live with it. Nothing is guaranteed, whether you have cancer or not. The good thing about cancer is that it reminds me to not push off to tomorrow what I can do today."

She seemed surprised by my candor, then relieved. This wasn't just her doctor speaking—it was someone who understood her fear from the inside out. We spent the next half hour talking not just about the results of her mammogram and how she was tolerating endocrine therapy but about how to navigate the space between vigilance and paranoia and steps she could take to thrive.

As for me, I still practice medicine and treat breast cancer patients, but I no longer define myself by the number of patients I see. I'm learning that it is okay to value and prioritize family time and getting better at protecting that time. Have I reviewed my monthly productivity figures? No. Do I want to serve on a hospital committee? No. Can we double book you? No. Am I available to peer review a paper for publication? No. I used to have a really hard time saying no because I was so worried about what others would think of me; but cancer has released me from these chains and given me the ability to live a life free of guilt and fear of repercussion.

I know where my priorities lie now and can better protect them by clearly defining my boundaries. And because I'm not overwhelmed by my clinic schedule, I'm able to see my patients differently now—with more empathy, more specificity, more awareness of both the science and the soul of healing. I continue to strive to provide excellent care but now understand that excellence requires that I support the whole person through their journey.

My sons watch me navigate this new normal. They've learned their own lessons about resilience, about showing up, about finding strength in vulnerability. Nathan still asks if I'm going to die sometimes, but now we can talk about fear without being consumed by it. Sam has learned to push through discomfort, to show up even when it's hard. James has grown into a young man who understands that strength and sensitivity can coexist. My ordinary moments now feel precious, and my fear now serves as a reminder to take nothing for granted and to live every day with gratitude and kindness.

Conclusion

BEGINNING AGAIN

The morning routine looks different now. Instead of screaming "Five minutes!" while frantically herding children toward the door, our day starts with a quieter rhythm.

Water bottles filled with ice water still appear on the counter, some habits of love don't change, but now my boys manage their own timing. James heads to his car by 6:45AM. Before he leaves, I kiss him on the cheek and remind him that I love him. Sam announces when it's time to head to the car as Nathan double-checks his face is clean. They both say, "I love you, Mom," before leaving the house. Not because they have to but because they want to. Because we've all learned that little moments matter and that words of love shouldn't wait.

The practice has changed too. Not the protocols or the advice I give but how I give it. Each patient gets more than medical guidance; they get specific strategies, concrete steps, real understanding. When they worry about symptoms, I listen differently. When they struggle with side effects, I offer solutions I've learned both as a doctor and as a survivor.

Working less isn't a sign of weakness; it's a choice for quality over quantity. The new full-time partner we brought in at our practice means I can leave early when I want to. I can prioritize being present over being productive. My worth isn't measured in the number of patients I see but in the depth of care I can provide.

I'm not going to sugarcoat it: Cancer changes you—not just physically but in every way that matters. You can't go back to who you were before diagnosis, before treatment, before understanding how quickly life can change. But maybe you can become someone better: more present, more compassionate, more alive to each moment.

And maybe that's the most important lesson of all: In the end, it's not just about surviving cancer. It's about living life—really living it—with all the wisdom, grace, and joy we can muster. Not despite our scars but because of them, and not despite our fears but alongside them.

This is what healing really looks like: it's not a return to what was, but an evolution into what can be.

About the Author

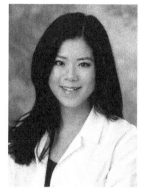

D r. Catherine Sue Hwang is a board-certified radiation oncologist that specializes in the treatment of breast cancer at the AdventHealth Cancer Institute in Orlando, Florida. She has dedicated her career to building its breast cancer program in Central Florida and has established herself as one of the leading breast radiation oncologists in the area. She serves as the Section Leader of Breast Radiation Oncology at the AdventHealth Cancer Institute and is an Associate Professor in Radiation Oncology at the University of Central Florida College of Medicine.

Since being diagnosed with breast cancer, she has developed a deeper understanding of the physical, psychological and social challenges associated with the disease. During treatment, she launched an Instagram page **@breast_cancer_360** to document her journey, increase breast cancer awareness, and discuss treatment related issues that many patients feel are overlooked. She first shared her doctor-patient experience in an essay published in the Huffington Post and soon found herself with a publishing deal to further share her journey. She has already started working on her next passion project which is tentatively titled: A How To Guide to Survivorship.

A free ebook edition is available with the purchase of this book.

To claim your free ebook edition:

1. Visit MorganJamesBOGO.com
2. Sign your name CLEARLY in the space
3. Complete the form and submit a photo of the entire copyright page
4. You or your friend can download the ebook to your preferred device

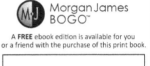

Morgan James BOGO™

A **FREE** ebook edition is available for you or a friend with the purchase of this print book.

CLEARLY SIGN YOUR NAME ABOVE

Instructions to claim your free ebook edition:
1. Visit MorganJamesBOGO.com
2. Sign your name CLEARLY in the space above
3. Complete the form and submit a photo of this entire page
4. You or your friend can download the ebook to your preferred device

Print & Digital Together Forever.

Snap a photo

Free ebook

Read anywhere

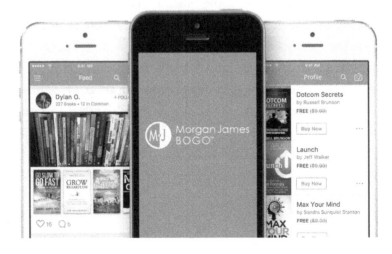